Down Syndrome across the Life Span

Down Syndrome across the Life Span

Edited by

MONICA CUSKELLY, ANNE JOBLING

University of Queensland

and

SUSAN BUCKLEY

University of Portsmouth

WHURR PUBLISHERS
LONDON AND PHILADELPHIA

First published 2002 by
Whurr Publishers Ltd
19b Compton Terrace, London N1 2UN, England
325 Chestnut Street, Philadelphia PA19106, USA

British Library Cataloguing in Publication Data

A catalogue record for this book is available from the
British Library.

ISBN 1 86156 230 6

Printed and bound in the UK by Athenaeum Press Limited,
Gateshead, Tyne & Wear.

Contents

Contributors

Gillian Bird, Director of Consultancy and Education, Down Syndrome Educational Trust, The Sarah Duffen Centre, Southsea, UK.

Sandra Bochner, Honorary Associate, School of Education, Macquarie University, Sydney, Australia.

Verity Bottroff, Senior Lecturer, and Associate Dean, School of Special Education and Disability Studies, Flinders University, Adelaide, Australia.

Anna Bower, Honorary Research Associate, Fred and Eleanor Schonell Special Education Research Centre, School of Education, University of Queensland, Brisbane, Australia.

Roy I. Brown, Professor Emeritus, Educational Psychology, University of Calgary; Foundation Professor, and Former Dean, School of Special Education and Disability Studies, Flinders University, Adelaide, Australia.

Sue Buckley, Director of Research and Training, Down Syndrome Educational Trust, The Sarah Duffen Centre, Southsea, UK.

Eddie Bullitis, School of Special Education and Disability Studies, Flinders University, Adelaide, Australia.

Sue Cairns, Lifestart Early Intervention Program, Turramurra, New South Wales, Australia.

David Chant, Associate Professor, Department of Psychiatry, University of Queensland, Brisbane, Australia.

Romeo Chua, Associate Professor, School of Human Kinetics, University of British Columbia, Vancouver, British Columbia, Canada.

Anna Contardi, Associazione Italiana Persone Down, Roma, Italy.

Cliff Cunningham, Visiting Professor, Health and Human Sciences, John Moores University, Liverpool, UK.

Monica Cuskelly, Co-Director, Down Syndrome Research Program, Fred and Eleanor Schonell Special Education Research Centre, Senior Lecturer, School of Education, University of Queensland, Brisbane, Australia.

Vicky Duffield, School of Special Education and Disability Studies, Flinders University, Adelaide, Australia.

Digby Elliott, Professor, Department of Kinesiology, McMaster University, Hamilton, Ontario, Canada.

Sheila Glenn, Professor, Health and Human Sciences, John Moores University, Liverpool, UK.

Loretta Giorcelli, Visiting Professor, San Francisco State University and Honorary Fellow, University of Western Sydney, Sydney, New South Wales, Australia.

Jan Gothard, Senior Lecturer, History Programme, Murdoch University, Murdoch, Western Australia, Australia.

John Grantley, Lecturer, School of Special Education and Disability Studies, Flinders University, Adelaide, Australia.

Alan Hayes, Professor of Early Childhood, School of Education, Macquarie University, Sydney, Australia

Matthew Heath, Assistant Professor, Department of Kinesiology, University of Indiana, Indiana, USA.

Anne Jobling, Co-Director, Down Syndrome Research Program, Fred and Eleanor Schonell Special Education Research Centre, Senior Lecturer, School of Education, University of Queensland, Brisbane, Australia.

Margaret Kyrkou, Medical Practitioner, Health and Education Service, School of Special Education and Disability Studies, Flinders University, Adelaide, Australia.

Brian K.V. Maraj, Assistant Professor, Perceptual Motor Behaviour Laboratory, Faculty of Physical Education and Recreation, University of Alberta, Edmonton, Alberta, Canada.

Roy McConkey, Professor of Learning Disability, School of Health Sciences, University of Ulster, Northern Ireland.

Karen B. Moni, Director, LATCH-ON, Fred and Eleanor Schonell Special Education Research Centre, Lecturer, School of Education, University of Queensland, Brisbane, Australia.

Susanne Muirhead, Registered Clinical Counsellor (Private Practice) British Columbia, Canada.

Lynne Outhred, Senior Lecturer, School of Education, Macquarie University, Sydney, Australia.

Moira Pieterse, Formerly Director, Down Syndrome Program, School of Education, Macquarie University, Sydney, Australia.

Shannon D. Robertson, Assistant Professor, Department of Exercise Science and Physical Education, Arizona State University, Arizona, USA.

Eric A. Roy, Department of Kinesiology and Psychology, University of Waterloo, Ontario, Canada.

Dominic A. Simon, Post-Doctoral Fellow, Department of Kinesiology, McMaster University, Hamilton, Ontario, Canada.

Judy Thornley, School of Special Education and Disability Studies, Flinders University, Adelaide, Australia.

Robin Treloar, Lifestart Early Intervention Program, Turramurra, New South Wales, Australia.

Christina E. van Kraayenoord, Director, Fred and Eleanor Schonell Special Education Research Centre, Senior Lecturer, School of Education, University of Queensland, Brisbane, Australia.

Daniel J. Weeks, Associate Professor, School of Kinesiology, Simon Fraser University, Vancouver, British Columbia, Canada.

Harold Weinberg, School of Kinesiology, Simon Fraser University, Vancouver, British Columbia, Canada.

Timothy N. Welsh, McMaster University, Hamilton, Ontario, Canada.

Jennifer G Wishart, Professor of Special Education, Moray House Institute of Education, University of Edinburgh, Edinburgh, U.K.

Kim Zeibarth, Guidance Officer, Education Queensland, Brisbane, Australia.

Preface

The 7th World Congress on Down syndrome was held in Sydney, Australia, in March 2000. The Congress is held approximately every four years and brings together researchers, professionals, parents, and lately, adults with Down syndrome from around the world. Contributors from 11 countries participated in the conference, discussing a diverse set of issues and presenting information on a range of research projects, interventions and services that had been developed with the aim of enhancing the lives of individuals with Down syndrome and of their families. Participants in the Congress came from an even larger number of countries and provided a lively discussion of the material presented in the various sessions.

It can be difficult to strike the right balance when organizing a conference that will include parents, professionals, and researchers as both presenters and audience. Each has different needs, expectations and background experiences, and understandings. There is a commonality, however, in the desire to improve understanding, and thus the lives, of individuals with Down syndrome and their families. The same dilemma occupied the editors of this collection.

The chapters presented in this book were collected together in order to provide readers with an introduction to some of the major issues confronting practitioners at this time. Not all areas of importance to those interested in Down syndrome have been included. Nevertheless, it is to be hoped that readers find some new insights in the material included here. The editors invited contributions from some of the individuals and groups who presented at the conference and the resulting book contains chapters from writers from four Australian states as well as from Canada, England, Iran, Italy, Northern Ireland, and Scotland. The dilemma alluded to above was resolved, at least in part, by including both researchers and practitioners in the contributors to the book, some of whom are also family of individuals with Down syndrome.

The content of the chapters covers a broad range of topics but there is a slight preponderance of chapters that focus on issues relevant to adults with

Down syndrome. This makes the book a very timely publication, as there is a growing recognition that our understanding of the needs, experiences, and desires of adults with Down syndrome is rather limited. As noted above, some of the chapters have been prepared by groups of researchers – one of the aims of the conference was to gather together research groups from across the world and to have them present an overview of their work. This has resulted in some chapters that briefly describe a number of research projects, rather than providing a more detailed report, although in these instances an overarching focus is clearly apparent. The editors have written a short introduction to each section of the book, at times to draw out themes and elsewhere to consider the implications of the work presented in the following chapters.

The organizing committee of the conference wished to include those with Down syndrome in the Congress and, to this end, involved a number of individuals in presentations to the entire audience as well as developing a parallel programme for adults with Down syndrome. This programme comprised seminars and workshops, in some cases delivered by individuals with Down syndrome, in addition to a social programme. The 'place' of individuals with Down syndrome in families, schools, communities, and in research, and the presentation of information about the lives of those with Down syndrome is a recurring theme throughout these chapters.

The final words of this preface belong to some of the people with Down syndrome who attended the Congress. The first is a record of a conversation between Luke Campbell and his mother.

Q: What kind of thing do you remember from the Down syndrome Congress at Darling Harbour, Luke?

A: You learn health. About anger and fear. How to be good and bad. Enjoy everyday life. If you are bad, no presents. If you're good, you get presents.

Q: You had a workshop on decision-making. What did you understand about that?

A: Someone in your head tells you what is good things to do and bad things. You walk your own path.

Q: At night after the second day, when you had the workshop on decision-making, poetry and about independence and joining in community things, you said to me 'Life is hard'. Was there anything in particular made you think that?

A: I felt scared and frightened about life. I felt good at the end of the Congress. Good to know how your brain works.

Luke Campbell

The workshops for people with Down syndrome were great. They were about friendships, feelings, keeping safe and decision-making for independence.

Linda Katuna-Rich

We talked about healthy food and watched videos. We talked about friends and drinking, when it is good for you and when it was bad for you.

Anne Power

I attended some workshops, and I enjoyed the Harbour cruise very much. But the highlight was the Congress dinner with live entertainment. It was really fantastic.

Caroline Brunner

The people with Down syndrome went along as well. We all got together – a special kind of people – once in our lifetime – to have fun.

Kylie Scott

Section 1
Views of self

Introduction

The chapter by Jan Gothard contained in this section breaks new ground for a publication such as this, coming as it does from the pen of an historian. Contributors to books on Down syndrome are more usually written by psychologists, educators, speech and language therapists, or those from the medical profession. As an historian Jan Gothard has used an approach to 'data gathering' which has enabled an aspect of the experience of Down syndrome that is usually presumed to be inaccessible to be presented. In her chapter she explicates her own decision-making as she approached her task of collecting the stories of adults with Down syndrome. The final product of this exploration was a project that gave skills to the individuals with Down syndrome to express their own perspectives.

Other chapters in this book, most particularly that by Muirhead (Chapter 12), also challenge the negative stereotypes that commonly surround individuals with Down syndrome. Both Gothard and Muirhead have used less traditional ways of collecting information and both force an examination of more commonly used methods.

Gothard leaves unresolved one of the most interesting aspects of the journey she describes – that is her frustration at the failure of the participants of her study to confirm for her the discrimination she believes they experience in their day-to-day lives. This impasse further highlights the relatively unexplored area of the emotional and social experiences of individuals with Down syndrome. We might hope that Gothard's chapter will ignite interest in this area, as well as suggest some ways of collecting authentic information.

CHAPTER 1
Beyond the myths: representing people with Down syndrome

JAN GOTHARD

Background

This chapter stems from my dual capacity as an historian and as the parent of Madeleine, an eight-year-old girl with Down syndrome. It is also partly autobiographical; my interest in disability and my work in the area are precisely as old as my daughter. The particular focus of this chapter is the way in which people with Down syndrome are represented, by themselves, as well as by others. The chapter outlines work still incomplete and seeks to show how my approach to representing people with Down syndrome has been illuminated and enhanced by my own reflections on my work and by the writings of others. Dealing initially with an oral history project of interviewing people with Down syndrome and their families, the chapter goes on to chart the growth of my belief that there are other, more powerful ways of representing people with Down syndrome. It concludes by arguing that, as important as representing people with Down syndrome is, facilitating self-representation is more important. Disability is discursively constructed and representations of individuals with Down syndrome, particularly from older and historical sources, can be a powerful vehicle for fostering negative responses and creating damaging stereotypical attitudes. Equally, they can promote positive attitudes and approaches. From this point of view, the most powerful contemporary representations are undoubtedly those produced by people with Down syndrome themselves.

Before my daughter was born, her father and I had had only extremely limited contact with people with any kind of intellectual disability. As is the case for most people outside the area, our ideas about Down syndrome had been quietly shaped by images from literature and the media, and by ignorance. Too often these things go together. Fay Weldon's book *Darcy's Utopia*, provides a telling example of some of the material in circulation which does so much to fashion our images and our ignorance about disabilities such as Down syndrome.

> I think about my friend Erin, as I often do. She has a Down's syndrome baby. We all knew it would be disastrous; we foretold that her husband would walk out, that her other children would suffer: we saw she was the only one of the family unit who couldn't bear not to see the fruit of her womb, however sour, ripen, drop and live. And that's how it turned out: the child, now twelve, is badly retarded, Erin is no more than its nurse; she manages without a husband, her other children are spiteful and embarrassed. Erin talks about the joy the mindless child brings her – well, so it may, but her love for it has been most destructive for others. Left to us, friends and family, we would have said no, Erin, sorry, not for you. This baby you insist on having keeps other babies out, ones which won't cause this distress to you and yours. Just not this one; Erin, try again.
>
> (Weldon, 1990: 140)

Once our daughter was born, my partner and I set out to find out more about Down syndrome and we were amazed at the legacy of historical ignorance we encountered. This related not simply to Down syndrome but to the whole field of disability. Fay Weldon might have been bad enough, but once we started delving into historical material, it quickly grew worse. Works such as Crookshank's *The Mongol in our Midst*, written in 1924, and Tredgold's 1908 classic *Mental Deficiency* (still in circulation and in its 10th edition in 1963), made us aware of how far ideas about people with intellectual disability had progressed but – thanks to Fay Weldon and others – we felt there was still ground to cover. We believed that

> the 'truth' of contemporary ideas about intellectual disability, while it produces better outcomes for people with intellectual disabilities than [earlier views], is still contingent on perception, interpretation and, above all, on the operation of the language through which humans think about the world.
>
> (Cocks and Allen, 1996: 283)

My partner channelled his intellectual energy into co-editing a history of intellectual disability in Western Australia, *Under Blue Skies* (Cocks, Fox, Brogan and Lee, 1996), while I drew on my experience as a practitioner of oral history. I knew my own life was nothing like the life Fay Weldon had suggested was in store for the parents of a child with Down syndrome and I wanted to understand more about other people's experiences. I wanted to know what life was like for individuals with Down syndrome. I wanted to confront some of the myths about Down syndrome and, perhaps idealistically, to be part of a process of debunking them. With the support of the Down Syndrome Association of Western Australia (DSAWA), I started work.

The original intention was to produce a book based on oral interviews and complementary research. From this emerged a scheme for a professionally produced photographic exhibition, drawing on themes important in the lives of families and individuals with Down syndrome. Finally a website was created to enable these photographs and associated material to be accessed more widely. The interview-based book, meanwhile, is on hold.

In retrospect, the process seems quite clear cut but in fact the path leading from the intended outcome of an interview-based book, to a photographic exhibition and website, was by no means straightforward and was littered with realizations about the implications of the work being undertaken. These issues will be addressed in the remainder of this chapter.

Limitations of the oral history approach

The starting point for this project was a series of interviews with the parents of people with Down syndrome. My agenda was clear; it was quite explicitly a bid to counter the Fay Weldonesque image of people with Down syndrome as 'mindless', their parents as 'little more than nurses', their siblings as soured and embittered. Certainly I had no difficulty in that task. But the intention was also to focus on the experience of *having* Down syndrome: how people with Down syndrome felt; how they were treated; what their expectations were; what difficulties they had encountered, if any, which they could attribute to their disability. I approached these issues in the broader context of finding out how young adults with Down syndrome lived their lives. And what I found was how very like, in many ways, the lives of my interviewees were to those of their peers who did not have a disability. Social interaction, recreation, education and training, relationships, work and family were the main foci of their lives. There were areas in which there were clear differences, largely associated with independence (driving cars featured strongly here) and leaving home (all my interviewees so far were living at home with their parents). On the whole, however, my interviews have reinforced the realization Jan Walmsley noted in other researchers: 'being a person with a learning disability is most akin to being a human being' (Walmsley, 1995: 72). At least, that was how my informants related their lives.

The question of the impact of having Down syndrome (a major focus of interest for me) I approached both obliquely and more directly, but my questioning seldom evoked the responses I had been expecting. Some informants were evidently surprised at my approach and politely expressed the view that the treatment they received and their relations with other people were 'normal'. Yet interviews also elicited this kind of story:

Interviewer: Can you tell me more about your sport?
Adam: I do swimming; I used to do netball . . . and badminton . . . and bowling . . . everything. My favourite is swimming. I was doing overarm, breaststroke, and . . . oh, and butterfly. Bowling is full of fun, and . . . I used to go bowling with a group of friends . . . It was fun.
                 Well, I used to play netball with a group, and . . . I didn't like it very much. I feel . . . left out, 'cause . . . they pushed me away. Well I felt . . . they were teasing me . . . talking behind my back . . . That really annoyed me . . . That's all.
Interviewer: So you stopped?
Adam: Yes.

When pressed further, however, Adam did not see this treatment as a possible function of his having Down syndrome. There are a number of issues to resolve here.

In the United Kingdom, Aull Davies and Jenkins (1997) have researched the 'significant incongruence' they had observed in a group of young adults with learning difficulties, between their 'categorical identity as someone with learning difficulties and their self-identity': in other words, their understandings of themselves did not take into account the fact that they had a disability. Aull Davies and Jenkins attribute this to the fact that the families of the 60 individuals in their group had evidently avoided any discussion with them relating to disability, one set of parents going so far as to black out all reference to Down syndrome in a press article relating to their son. This was certainly not the case with my interviewees.

Adam had represented the state on several occasions in swimming and athletics and had a fistful of medals as testimony to his sporting prowess in 'special' sporting competition; and the mother of another young woman assured me her daughter would tell me 'in no uncertain terms' what it was like to have Down syndrome. (She didn't.) All of these individuals in any case, through their families, were members of the DSAWA. That was how I had contacted them, and their membership meant that these young adults had generally mixed socially with others with Down syndrome and certainly took active advantage of the recreational offerings made available through the DSAWA and other similar groups for people with disabilities. They all understood very clearly that they had Down syndrome and that this made them 'different': 'special'.

What their parents had tried to protect them from was the stigma associated with Down syndrome. In many ways they had been successful: for example, how many people with Down syndrome would have read Fay Weldon? Where they encountered images of Down syndrome it was more often in terms of positive media representations. The American television series *Life Goes On* was widely watched, and so too was the Australian television production *House Gang*, a series centred around a group house and featuring three young adults with Down syndrome as well as other characters with intellectual disability. They had been largely protected from the most negative aspects of the prevalent discourse associated with disability.

I also had to confront my own response to statements about the normality of the lives led by young adults with Down syndrome. I found myself here in the position Hamilton (1992) has discussed: interviewing people who did not acknowledge their own oppression. Why weren't they interested in telling the story I most wanted to hear? Like Hamilton, I found it almost impossible to divorce my questioning of people with Down syndrome from my own political and social understanding of their positions in society as a marginalized one. The sociologist Goodley has discussed this as it relates to interviewing people with learning difficulties, pointing out that in their questioning, when they focus on areas which are of greatest concern to them, researchers risk 'imposing their own assumptions, understanding and ambitions upon the stories that emerge' (1996: 345). This certainly meshed with my own experience.

Another associated issue was the veracity of accounts, for example, accounts of treatment that was 'normal'. Was the informant telling the truth? Here I felt more comfortable. Few oral historians believe that what they are uncovering is an unmediated truth; rather it is evidence of how one person perceives his or her experience and is prepared to communicate it. Dean and Foote Whyte (1995. Cited in Walmsley 1995: 74) point out that all accounts are revealing and that truth itself is not the issue. Yet I also wanted people with Down syndrome to acknowledge the negative aspects of their experience of disability. Interviewing did not enable me to tap into this.

Similar issues, familiar to all oral historians but reinforced in the case of people with an intellectual disability, relate to the material generated by an interview (Goodley, 1996; Walmsley, 1995). Once interviews have been produced, if the material is to be used by other people some process of transcription and editing is essential, for example in the extract from Adam's interview cited above. It has been widely argued that the process of transcribing and editing the stories generated by one culture so as to be accessible to people of another, can lead to re-readings, re-writings and ultimately corruption. (This is a subject of virulent debate in Australia where interviews with Aboriginal people are often transcribed for just that reason, to facilitate interpretation by another culture.) This is also true of reworking the words of people with Down syndrome, or indeed with any kind of developmental delay or learning difficulty. In the role of editor of memories, there is a danger of writing one's own stories rather than the informant's. Retelling, using extracts of interviews to make a point, undoubtedly misrepresents the narrative faculties of the person transcribed. (I have done precisely this in the example above, where Adam talks about his sporting interests.) This particular problem is heightened in the case of informants with underdeveloped literacy skills, especially amongst older informants with Down syndrome (Walmsley, 1995).

Oral history came into prominence in the 1960s and 1970s with the rise of the new social history, as a way of shifting the historical focus away from those with political power; hence it became the tool of people working in, for example, women's history, histories of race relations, and labour history. Oral history is understood as a process whereby historians could give back a voice to the powerless, to the historically inarticulate. However, the notion of 'inarticulate' is qualified; we still assume some degree of 'voice' on the part of the informant. Here we encounter Baron's 'paradox': 'those who most need to have their stories heard may be the least able to tell them' (Booth and Booth, 1996: 59).

Most people with Down syndrome can speak. Many, particularly younger people with Down syndrome, have had the benefit of early intervention and speech therapy, not to mention heightened expectations these days about their capacities. All these things were largely denied to people with Down syndrome less than a generation ago. Such people can be very articulate indeed. Indeed my own eight-year-old never stops talking. Their experiences are certainly worth recording and I have begun to do so. But to get a feel for what life was like, perhaps for people who were institutionalized, or even for those who stayed home but were given little access to education, who were assumed to have had, not simply an intellectual or learning disability but to be uninterested in and incapable of learning: capturing the recollections of those people is harder. How do we give voice to those people whose voices are so muted and muffled as to be almost literally inaudible?

These problems have been confronted by most oral historians working with people with intellectual disabilities and learning difficulties and – like me – oral historians have continued to pursue this method of recording aspects of the lives of their informants, on the grounds that any attempt is better than leaving this group of people entirely without voice. Booth and Booth (1996), Goodley (1996), Walmsley (1995) and the widely cited Fido and Potts (1989) all provide strong evidence that the difficulties, though real, can be surmounted.

Written representations

There are, of course, other models than the oral interview for recording the lives of people with Down syndrome. Most common are books written by parents on behalf of their children with Down syndrome; those by Espinas (1989), Hardie (1991), Rogers and Dolva (1998) and Kaly (1998) are all fairly typical examples and demonstrate an interesting international similarity in approach. One such book, Lloyd Clifford's *Three Loves* (1984), is introduced with these lines:

> The book I have written is an attempt to put into words, the thoughts, feelings, and understandings of a certain type of human being, viz – a mongol. As far as I am aware, not one of these happy people would be capable of putting into words, let alone writing down their story, as I have tried to do.

Not all parents' books share this disappointing perception of the capacities of their children and by association all people with Down syndrome, but certainly a number do.

Much more positively, in a 'parent' book of quite a different style, Michael Berube (1998) looks forward to the time when people with Down syndrome will not need books like his, written on their behalf. There are already at least two English-language autobiographies in circulation; the book *The World of Nigel Hunt* (Hunt, 1967) is a classic and, more recently, we have the American publication *Count Us In!* (Kingsley and Levitz, 1994) written by two young men with Down syndrome. Such publications, however, are still rare. Their existence is testimony to the often unrecognized potential of people with Down syndrome; but, while they are likely to increase in number as opportunities available to people with Down syndrome improve, they are unlikely to become commonplace.

Alternative modes of representation

If words have limitations, can we move beyond them? Recognizing some of the limitations of the oral history approach, not least the practical issue of the time required to mount such a project and make the material accessible, the DSAWA decided to try. We set out to counter some of the widely circulated myths in currency about Down syndrome through the medium of photography. Myths such as 'all mothers of children with Down syndrome are old', 'all children with Down syndrome look alike', 'people with Down syndrome cannot keep learning beyond a certain level', 'all people with Down syndrome are constantly happy and love music' and 'people with Down syndrome cannot mix beyond their own kind': these were all confronted and debunked in a series of commissioned photographs taken by professional photographer Mona Neumann. These photographs were then displayed in an exhibition which was open to the public for about four months, during which time it was visited by more than 8000 people. At the initiative of the Museum of Western Australia, the photographic exhibition was then put on permanent and international display as the museum's first public access exhibition website.

Excited as we were about the potential of the photographic exhibition, the DSAWA was still aware of some of the limitations of this approach. As is evident in texts such as Crookshank (1924) and Tredgold (1908), photography can reinforce the negative. The medical model of disability, in particular, has been served only too well by images from these sorts of sources. One such photograph depicts people with Down syndrome held rigidly before the camera, with an attendant's hands clamped firmly and visibly on each subject's ears to prevent movement. In another image, a person with Down syndrome has his/her mouth held wide open with the tongue pulled out by instrument, to allow the camera to view the lines and marking sometimes said to be typical of the 'patient' with Down syndrome. Yet another photograph shows a young 'Mongol' boy sitting in lotus position, his 'Orientalism' inscribed on his body for the camera to see.

More recently, people with disabilities have begun to appear in photographic collections other than the medical, and as this has occurred, so too have critics begun to analyse. Diane Arbus (1990), 'the photographer of freaks', with her work on people with Down syndrome (her 'retardees') and David Hevey's (1992, 1997) savage indictment of her approach are amongst the best known. Hevey has also cast a critical eye over charity images of people with disability and although we were then unaware of Hevey's work, the DSAWA was eager not to add to the genre of people with disabilities either as 'basket cases' requiring sympathy and a cash handout, or as 'supercrips' (Hevey, 1992; Corbett and Ralph, 1994). Thus our exhibition focused on addressing myths which had wide currency and on dismissing them through photographs of people with Down syndrome going about their normal lives.

Nonetheless, creating even positive images about people with Down syndrome as the object of the camera's gaze, or as the object of the interviewer's questionings, was not enough. It became important to move away from that objectification of people with Down syndrome to have them create their own stories, to represent themselves. As I had believed when conducting my interviews, and as Hevey himself has written, 'I have yet to meet the disabled person who was not aware more or less, of his or her oppression' (Hevey, 1992: 2). Capturing their awareness of that oppression, as I had largely failed to do through interviews, and permitting people with Down syndrome to 'work through the . . . desire to fight back' (Hevey, 1992: 2) became our next objective. Thus we moved on, from people with Down syndrome as objects to people

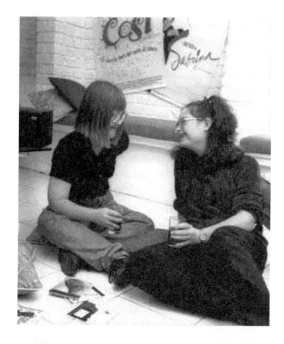

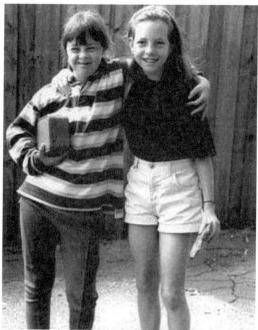

Some of my best friends have Down syndrome . . . and some of them don't.
© Down Syndrome Association of Western Australia (Inc.)

with Down syndrome as photographers, by encouraging young adults with Down syndrome to create their own photographic statements about their lives.

Through structured group workshops, participants discussed issues important to them, such as sexuality, personal relations, and independence. Then, using the skills learned through the photographic workshop, they collectively created photographic images to reinforce the themes of their discussions. Some of these photographs were then displayed as part of a public exhibition, and were later used on the website. (This workshop approach was also used to generate scripts for the SBS television series *House Gang*: Meekosha and Dowse, 1997.)

It's a commonplace that every picture tells a story, that a picture is worth a thousand words; but it's also true that a picture can tell a thousand stories to a thousand different viewers. In the context of the workshop, the group wanted to tell very particular stories through their images. For that reason, each image was associated with some brief text. The text was not written by workshop participants, but emerged as a result of conversations within the group, as a natural part of the workshopping process. Reproduced here are some of the results, with the accompanying text.

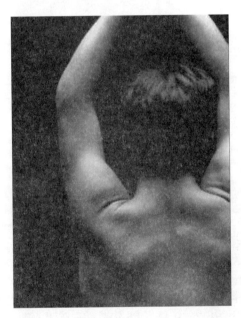

My body is beautiful. © Down Syndrome Association of Western Australia (Inc.)

One of Justin's passions is bodybuilding. As people with Down syndrome are often aware, some older stereotypes of people with Down syndrome caricature them as shambling and physically unattractive. Justin's body is beautiful by any standards.

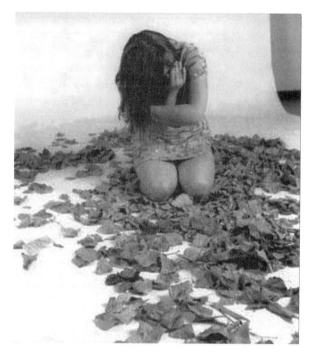

I often feel lonely. © Down Syndrome Association of Western Australia (Inc.)

Wanting to protect those we love is natural, but protection can sometimes lead to cocooning, with a much-loved child cut off from the rough and tumble of everyday life. The consequences can strike home as people reach teen years and adulthood; young people growing up can experience love and protection as loneliness and isolation. While this certainly isn't always the case, loneliness can be part of the experience of growing up with Down syndrome. 'Letting go' of their children with Down syndrome and allowing them 'the dignity of risk' may be one of the most difficult issues parents have to confront.

Conclusions

What are the implications of this process for representing lives? I am not suggesting that oral historians all trade in their Sonys for Leicas, their tape recorders for cameras, but this project does have both a methodological and ethical resonance when we consider ways of recording the lives of people with learning difficulties. It may be that the very idea of 'giving a voice' to people with an intellectual disability, though well intended, is in itself patronizing. It may be that the sorts of questions I was asking in my interviews – 'What do people with Down syndrome have to say about themselves, and why?' – are not the appropriate ones. Teaching skills, and then leaving those who have them to record what they will of their lives – through photography,

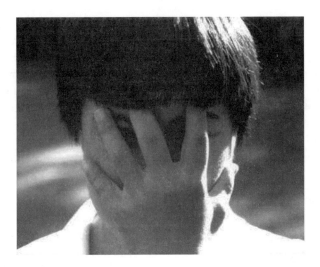

Give me the chance to see the world my own way! © Down Syndrome Association of Western Australia (Inc.)

> Like Melissa, many people with Down syndrome find it frustrating to have their different life experiences overlooked or denied in a society that assumes that all people are similarly 'able'. For minority groups, finding an appropriate means of self-expression can be particularly important. Some people with Down syndrome have chosen to write about how they see their world. Drama is also an important means of self-expression. For others, art and photography are excellent alternative means through which to present their views. The photographic workshop that enabled the production of many of these photographs is an excellent example of this.

through workshopping interviews, whatever – may be one way around that problem. In the UK, family history skills are already being taught to people with learning difficulties through the Open University (Open University, 1996). In the Australian context, the Western Australian venture into a group photography workshop, the Exhibition and the website, is, I believe, the first major attempt to encourage people with Down syndrome to represent their own lives, and to give then a major public vehicle for circulating their ideas.

The images which emerged from the DSAWA workshops were not created by people who came together with any political interests or with the specific intention of self-empowerment. They were part of the group because their parents encouraged them to be, for social and recreational reasons and to acquire useful skills. The workshop photographs are at one level the product of discussions led by outsiders who did not have Down syndrome, which focused specifically on the question: 'What is it like to have Down syndrome?' Left entirely to themselves, the workshop participants might well have preferred to use their newly acquired skills to take photographs of architecture, street scenes, animals or beaches. There was still an outside hand directing the process. Nonetheless, the photographic images were all ultimately generated by people who have Down syndrome. While the movement for self-advocacy grows, these tentative steps towards self-representation are surely an important beginning. These images can be read as poignant and powerful political statements about what it means to be a young adult with Down syndrome: statements which focus on the lived experience of disability in ways which my interviews could not.

References

Arbus D (1990) diane arbus. London: Bloomsbury Press.

Aull Davies C, Jenkins R (1997) 'She has different fits to me': how people with learning difficulties see themselves. Disability and Society 12: 95–109.

Berube M (1998) Life as We Know It: A Father, a Family and an Exceptional Child. New York: Vintage Books.

Booth T, Booth W (1996) Sounds of silence: narrative research with inarticulate subjects. Disability and Society 11: 55–69.

Clifford L (1984) Three Loves. Somerset: Clifford Davis.

Cocks E, Allen M (1996) Discourses of disability. In Cocks E, Fox C, Brogan M, Lee M (Eds) Under Blue Skies: The Social Construction of Intellectual Disability in Western Australia. Perth: Edith Cowan University. pp 282–318.

Cocks E, Fox C, Brogan M, Lee M (Eds) Under Blue Skies: The Social Construction of Intellectual Disability in Western Australia. Perth: Edith Cowan University.

Corbett J, Ralph S (1994) Empowering adults: the changing image of charity advertising. Australian Disability Review 1: 5–13.

Crookshank FG (1924) The Mongol in our Midst. London: Kegan Paul.

Dean J, Foot Whyte W (1995) How do you know if the informant is telling the truth? In Bynner J, Stribley K (Eds) Social Research: Principles and Procedures. London: Longman.

Espinas J (1989) Your Name is Olga (1986). Translated by Pamela Waley. London: Unwin Hyman Ltd.

Fido R, Potts M (1989) 'It's not true what was written down!' Experiences of life in a mental handicap institution. Oral History (Autumn): 31–34.

Goodley D (1996) Tales of hidden lives: a critical examination of life history research with people who have learning difficulties. Disability and Society 11: 333–48.

Hamilton P (1992) 'Inventing the self': oral history as autobiography. In Donaldson I, Read P, Walter J (Eds) Shaping Lives: Reflections of Autobiography. Canberra: Humanities Research Centre, ANU. pp 110–16.

Hardie S (1990) Why me? 'Autobiography' of Sheenagh Hardie, a Down's Syndrome Girl, assisted by her parents Helen and Alastair Hardie. London: Excalibur Press.

Hevey D (1992) The Creatures Time Forgot: Photography and Disability Imagery. London: Routledge.

Hevey D (1997) The Enfreakment of Photography. In Davis LJ (Ed) The Disability Studies Reader. London: Routledge. pp 332–47.

Hunt N (1967) The World of Nigel Hunt: The Diary of a Mongoloid Youth. Beaconsfield: Darwen Finlayson.

Kaly S (1998) Down Syndrome: How One Family Coped with the Challenge. Sydney: Wild and Woolley.

Kingsley J, Levitz M (1994) Count Us In: Growing Up with Down Syndrome. San Diego: Harcourt Brace and Company.

Meekosha H, Dowse L (1998) Distorting images, invisible images: gender, disability and the media. Media International Australia 84: 91–101.

Open University (1996) K503: Working as Equal People. Milton Keynes: Open University.

Rogers C, Dolva G (1998) Karina Has Down Syndrome. Lismore: Southern Cross University Press.

Tredgold AF (1908) Mental Deficiency. London: Bailliere (10th ed: 1963).

Walmsley J (1995) Life history interviews with people with learning disabilities. Oral History 23 (Spring): 71–7.

Weldon F (1990) Darcy's Utopia. London: Collins.

SECTION 2

MOTIVATION, LEARNING AND

SELF-REGULATION IN YOUNG CHILDREN

Introduction

Both chapters in this section deal with motivation in young children with Down syndrome, and both also present additional information which contributes to our understanding of the relevance of motivation to the lives of individuals with Down syndrome. In this commentary, however, we shall initially discuss the motivational research before considering the other material contained within the papers.

Jennifer Wishart reports on a longitudinal study where children were repeatedly presented with object permanence tasks of increasing difficulty. Initial findings suggested children with Down syndrome were able to successfully complete the easier versions of the task at an age that was earlier than had previously been thought possible. Later attempts to elicit this behaviour were often met with refusals to participate, however. Difficult tasks were often refused or avoided. Wishart interprets her findings as indicating that young children with Down syndrome are less motivated to engage in activities that will promote their learning than are typically developing children. Sheila Glenn and Cliff Cunningham, on the other hand, report a study that found that young children with Down syndrome did not differ in mastery motivation from mental-age-matched peers who were developing typically, at most of the ages studied. There was, however, a difference at 12 months with children with Down syndrome displaying lower mastery than the comparison group.

Maternal responses to a questionnaire about mastery motivation contradicted the experimental findings reported by Glenn and Cunningham. Mothers of a child with Down syndrome reported reduced motivation in their children in comparison with the mothers of typically developing children. This reflects the findings of Wishart and makes it clear that we cannot be too quick to adopt the position that motivation is not a problem for children with Down syndrome. The developmental lag shown in the data reported by Glenn and Cunningham also requires consideration. Children with Down syndrome were showing similar changes in interests to the typically developing group, but these appeared at developmental ages that were six months behind their peers, suggesting an asynchrony between some elements of development. More work is required to understand the implications of these studies and to ascertain the most effective ways of keeping children with Down syndrome engaged with learning, in all its facets.

Wishart makes the case that children's partners in learning are likely to have an important role in developing or stifling motivation. Her research found that the stereotype of the child with Down syndrome was still very much a current view, even amongst those who would be thought to know better. Such views can only work against producing the most appropriate educational environment for children with Down syndrome. Finding the right balance between understanding the typical development of children with Down syndrome and the characteristics of the individual child can be a difficult challenge.

The second part of the Glenn and Cunningham chapter deals with an issue that is of concern to the parents of many adolescents with Down syndrome – talking to oneself. The editors have each had conversations about this behaviour with many a concerned parent, so it is gratifying to have data that can inform our response. Glenn and Cunningham argue convincingly that talking aloud to oneself is a developmental phenomenon which should cause little concern to parents when it occurs in an adolescent with Down syndrome as it is generally appropriate for developmental level. They suggest that parents focus on teaching their child where such behaviours should not occur (using the pragmatic yardstick of public places) rather than on trying to suppress the behaviour altogether. The authors draw the two studies together by presenting them within the framework of self-regulation, a framework that is likely to prove very productive in assisting the development of independence in those with Down syndrome. They make the interesting point that private speech is related to the development of the concept of self, a relatively overlooked aspect of development in those with Down syndrome.

Chapter 2
Learning in young children with Down syndrome: public perceptions, empirical evidence

Jennifer G Wishart

Many of the biggest obstacles faced by young children with Down syndrome in their everyday lives stem from their reduced ability to learn at the same rate and in the same way as other children. Many of these learning difficulties are biologically determined, the direct result on neurological development of the activity of excess genes on the third copy of chromosome 21. Gene therapy to counteract the adverse effects of some specific genetic disorders is already possible and in principle could at some point in the future be available for Down syndrome. This is clearly still a very long way off, however, and although genetic understanding is increasing at an astonishing rate, it is far from clear how great the practical benefits will be for those with developmental disabilities in which a large numbers of genes are known to be implicated, such as Down syndrome.

Not all of the factors influencing learning in children with Down syndrome are primarily biological, however. There are other obvious influences on the children's rates of developmental progress, not least the psychological environment in which they grow and learn and the ways in which their learning partners – parents, teachers and peers – support their efforts to learn. The evidence suggests that neither of these is currently as well tailored to meeting the special educational needs of children with Down syndrome as it might be, but also that both are open to change.

Providing a maximally supportive learning environment is obviously critical for children with Down syndrome. Developmental psychologists have a central role in identifying those environmental factors which support the learning process and those which do not, and it is from this disciplinary perspective that this chapter is written. It is based mainly on findings from a series of inter-linked investigations of cognitive and socio-cognitive development in children with Down syndrome which have been carried out in Edinburgh over the last 15 years or so and makes no claims to cover the wider literature on development in Down syndrome. This has been covered in several other books, including the excellent Cicchetti and Beeghly (1990) and Stratford and Gunn (1996).

Cognitive development in children with Down syndrome is often assumed to be simply a slowed-down version of normal development. Findings from the Edinburgh studies strongly suggest, however, that the process of development in Down syndrome is fundamentally different, both in its nature and course. If this is the case, then differences in the children's natural learning style, and in the routes by which their development progresses, will need to be taken into account in the design and delivery of early intervention and educational programmes if they these are to have any chance of achieving their aims.

Some of the data from the Edinburgh programme of longitudinal and cross-sectional studies have demonstrated that early ability in young children with Down syndrome can be surprisingly high (see e.g. Wishart, 1987, 1991, 1993; Franco and Wishart, 1995). It appears though that early successes are sometimes inadequately consolidated and consequently developmental progress often proves to be uneven. The precise mechanisms underlying this developmental instability are not yet fully understood, but it is likely that motivational deficits in the children themselves, coupled with low expectations in their partners in learning, play an important role in determining rates of development and final levels of achievement. Some of the motivational deficits seen in children with Down syndrome may stem from inherent differences in key brain structures but some may well be acquired, a by-product of often adverse learning experiences. For most of the children even fairly simple childhood skills can take a very long time to learn. It would be surprising if this did not impact unfavourably on the motivation to invest further effort in learning, although direct evidence of this interaction is not always easy to gather.

Learning in children with Down syndrome: fact and fiction

In trying to support children with Down syndrome in their learning, it is important to have some idea of the sort of ability levels they are likely to achieve. Many misconceptions and preconceptions exist in people's minds about the nature and extent of the difficulties Down syndrome can cause for those who have it. Although it is probably the best known of all of the learning disabilities, there are still more misconceptions about Down syndrome than about almost any other condition affecting children's mental development – not only amongst the general public but also within many of the professions that come into contact with children with Down syndrome. Ironically, most people probably now consider themselves to be much better informed about genetically-determined syndromes than preceding generations. Having some knowledge of the aetiology of conditions such as Down syndrome is commonplace and anyone now using the word 'mongol' in public would be likely to get very short shrift in most company. Images of attractive young people in parent-sponsored poster campaigns and exposure to actors with Down syndrome in high profile TV soaps have undoubtedly helped to dispel many of the negative views previously held by those with no personal contact with anyone with the syndrome. We need to consider carefully though just how deeply these changes in attitudes really go and how much they influence actual behaviour towards those with Down syndrome.

Findings from two of our studies have provided some information on public and professional expectations of children with Down syndrome and indicate that many misconceptions still run deep – and in some unexpected quarters. In the first study, we looked at attribution of a stereotyped personality to children with Down syndrome (Wishart and Johnston, 1990), and in the second, at the attitudes of trainee teachers towards educational inclusion for children with Down syndrome and their expectations of developmental potential in this particular group of children (Wishart and Manning, 1996). In the stereotyping study, we asked nine groups of adults with differing levels of experience and contact with children with Down syndrome – parents, teachers and students at a late stage in their professional training as doctors, health visitors and psychologists – to fill in a questionnaire telling us what they knew about Down syndrome as a condition and what they knew about children who had Down syndrome. They were asked to pick from a five-point bipolar rating scale those characteristics which they 'believed best describe the personality of DS children under 12 years of age'. The list contained 26 characteristics compiled from the literature on Down syndrome (e.g. outgoing/withdrawn; affectionate/undemonstrative); three of the 26 characteristics had 'ends' both of which had been described in the literature as stereotypical (e.g. docile/stubborn).

The task set was, of course, a trick one – there is no such thing as 'the' child with Down syndrome, whatever the age – but that did not stop virtually all of the sample from ticking one or other end of each of the paired characteristics. Statements like 'DS children are super to work with – such loving wee souls' were also readily entered in the box for additional comments at the end of the questionnaire. Only five highly experienced special school teachers irately returned the questionnaire and said it was impossible to fill in meaningfully. Mainstream primary teachers, teachers from integrated schools – with and without direct experience of working with children with Down syndrome – and the remaining special school teachers all returned completed questionnaires, as did the medical students, the psychology students and the health visitor trainees, all producing profiles which fitted well with the Down syndrome stereotype as portrayed in the literature. Surprisingly, mothers who had a child with Down syndrome also readily endorsed the stereotype, although to a lesser degree. Interestingly, and paradoxically, when given the opportunity to fill in two questionnaires, one for children with Down syndrome in general and one specifically in relation to their own child with Down syndrome, they attributed the stereotype more strongly to their own child. Mothers with children of a similar age, but without Down syndrome, were also happy to endorse the Down syndrome stereotype; when asked to fill in a second questionnaire in relation to typically developing 12-year-olds, however, all considered this an impossible task.

Clearly, children with Down syndrome are believed to have some common identity whereas ordinary children are considered to have distinctive, individual personalities. The fact that the stereotype endorsed was predominantly positive should not necessarily be taken as a positive finding. An 'easy' stereotype may result in unnecessarily low demands being made of children with Down syndrome, both in terms of effort and behaviour, and this cannot be beneficial in the long run. The one encouraging finding was that those adults with more frequent contact with children with Down syndrome were significantly less emphatic in their attribution of the stereotype than those with little contact. With the exception of those teachers already working with children with Down syndrome, however, it was surprising how few of the teachers, parents and trainee professionals in this study had had any personal experience of children with Down syndrome, whether in social or professional contexts. Both social and educational inclusion, it would seem, are much more spoken about than experienced.

The second study aimed to look more directly at what the next generation of teachers expects from young children with Down syndrome in terms of their developmental potential. Two hundred and thirty-one trainee teachers were asked their views on inclusive education and asked to assess the ages at which children with Down syndrome might achieve some specific developmental milestones (e.g. toilet training; simple reading and writing skills). The students were all in their third year of a four-year, university-based teacher training course in one of two United Kingdom institutions.

Findings were not encouraging. Only 13 per cent of the trainee teachers in this study indicated that they would welcome the opportunity to teach in an integrated setting and 96 per cent felt that their professional training to date had not prepared them for this challenge. As few were likely to get much more in the way of specialized input on meeting special educational needs in the remainder of their courses, this is of some concern – especially given the near unanimity in responses that this was the most important factor in determining whether integration would succeed or fail. No less discouraging were the respondents' expectations of developmental potential in children with Down syndrome. Estimates of age of likely achievement of each of the developmental milestones were typically pessimistic, suggesting ages higher than those reported in the developmental literature for Down syndrome. Most worrying were predictions of average life expectancy. Few respondents expected children with Down syndrome to survive beyond the age of 30 when in fact average life expectancy is now very little different from that for many of the rest of the population: 60 to 70 years (Baird and Sadovnik, 1988). Expectations of an abbreviated life span would seem bound to influence the skills are seen as important to acquire in the childhood years and it was not therefore surprising that many of the sample rated the benefits of inclusive education as being more social than educational.

Successfully educating children with special educational needs alongside their peers obviously depends heavily on the commitment of teachers to making it work, both in social and academic terms. There is much rhetoric in this area and a great deal of political and professional pressure on teachers to conform to the view that inclusive education is the only way forward. Teachers generally have little choice in the matter – and often very little advance notice that a child with special educational needs will be joining their class. Legislation, practice, resources, and training opportunities vary greatly across countries and, even within the same country, the implementation of inclusive education can often vary markedly in neighbouring regions. In 'flagship' schools, given ample resources, active experience of inclusion and investment in high-level professional development courses, there is some evidence that confidence levels of staff can be raised, positive attitudes fostered, and achievement levels raised (see e.g. Avramidis, Bayliss and Burden, 2000; Buckley and Bird, this volume). Findings from other recent studies (e.g. Forlin, 1995), however, suggest that direct experience of working with children with special educational needs in mainstream classrooms may actually lessen the enthusiasm of some teachers for inclusive education. There are a number of methodological issues to be addressed before a clearer picture will emerge and it would therefore be unsafe to conclude that time and experience will necessarily change the views of the trainee teachers sampled in our study. In the absence of specialist training or additional classroom resources, it is possibly unrealistic to expect that every teacher will feel competent to meet the challenge of teaching children who have a significant level of learning difficulty – and it is therefore unsurprising that few feel confident that they will easily be able to do so.

How do children with Down syndrome learn?

There is little doubt that if educational support is tailored to their specific educational needs, most children with Down syndrome will benefit greatly from their time spent at school. Some individual children progress to levels that would previously have been considered unattainable for anyone with Down syndrome but for the majority it is fair to say that acquiring everyday social and academic skills will still remain a very uphill task, no matter how skilled the teaching. Although little can currently be done about the harmful effects that the extra chromosome has on the children's ability to learn, there may nevertheless be ways to compensate for some of the resulting difficulties. In some of our studies, however, many of the children in fact seemed to go out of their way to *avoid* opportunities to learn. The greater their experience of learning, the more they seemed to rely on the help of other people, even when it was not needed, and the less they seemed willing to take the initiative in solving problems for themselves. Children with Down syndrome would sometimes seem to adopt an approach to learning that is far from productive, one that can actually make learning much harder than it really needs to be.

Why should this be? Looking at the likely learning histories of children with Down syndrome may provide some clues. All of the children come to learning with an inherent biological disadvantage: put simply, nature has denied them some of the basic neurological tools required for efficient learning. This in-built disadvantage can only be compounded by the adverse effects of the protracted nature of much of their learning. Repeated exposure to failure in new learning contexts and to the typically low expectations of their partners in learning must also make for a very difficult psychological environment in which to learn. Rates of progress fall increasingly behind those of age peers, a widening developmental gap which seems to be relatively unaffected by early intervention – despite the considerable parental and professional effort currently invested in such programmes (see e.g. Duffy, 1990; Wishart 1993, 1996, 1998).

Some of the data from our studies have highlighted just how quickly development in children with Down syndrome diverges from typical developmental pathways and one of the main aims of our research programme has been to try to pinpoint some of the factors underlying the decline in developmental rate apparently associated with the syndrome (see e.g. Carr, 1995).

Children in our studies have ranged in age from birth to 14 years, with numbers in specific studies varying from 10 to 50. In the longitudinal studies, data collection has extended from 1 to 5 years, depending on the age of children at entry and the nature of the questions being addressed by the specific study. In most studies, control groups of children without Down syndrome have also been tested in order to allow direct evaluation of difference versus delay theories. These typically developing children were matched with the children with Down syndrome on either chronological age or stage in development, depending on the focus of the particular study. It is apparent from some of the findings, however, that 'matching' is a somewhat misleading and sometimes meaningless concept when it comes to Down syndrome. Children with Down syndrome simply do not respond in test situations in the same way as ordinary children, even when they achieve similar 'scores'. Sometimes they do not even provide satisfactory matches for themselves. The content and the quality of responses in two identical, closely spaced testing sessions can often fluctuate greatly, with successes in a first session no longer being demonstrated in a second and with first session 'failures' miraculously turning into successes only a week or two later (Wishart and Duffy, 1990).

There is only space here to outline briefly data from one longitudinal study, a study of object concept development but the findings from this will point up some of the key features which appear to characterize early development in children with Down syndrome. The tasks set in these object concept studies - looking for a toy under one of two paper cups after a variety of hiding sequences - may seem far removed from the sorts of understanding young children might need in their everyday lives. However, these tasks tap abilities crucial to understanding the relationship between what we do and what happens in the world around us. We all have to learn at some point, for example, that objects exist independently of our actions and continue to exist even when we cannot see them or act upon them. We also have to learn that objects cannot be in two places at the one time and that they all have unique identities - two objects seen at different times may look identical, but they are not necessarily the same object - and so on. Without this knowledge, the world in which we live would be an unfathomable and very unpredictable place.

Thirty infants with Down syndrome took part in our longitudinal study of object concept development. Four different levels of tasks were used and testing sessions were fortnightly, with the same tester being used on all occasions. Although there was already evidence to suggest that children with Down syndrome would be likely to be considerably delayed in acquiring each of the stages in object concept development tapped by these tasks, we fortunately decided to try all levels of task with all children in all testing sessions, irrespective of current age.

Mean age of first success on each of the tasks turned out to be very encouraging. Although the children with Down syndrome took longer than control children to achieve their first success (4/4 correct searches on any given level of task, with success repeated in the following session), most nevertheless first succeeded at far younger ages than previous cross-sectional studies would have suggested were possible. On the second easiest of the four tasks, the AAB task, for example, mean age of first success was $7^3/_4$ months for the typically developing infants and $10^1/_2$ months for the infants with Down syndrome; with range of age of first success of $7^1/_4$–14 months in the Down syndrome group. The bottom line was that these infants with Down syndrome may on average have taken longer to achieve their first success on this particular task but the mean age at which they did so was not far off cross-sectional norms for age of acquisition of this stage in development (10 months). A small number of infants in fact succeeded at surprisingly early ages, a pattern also found in performance on the higher-level tasks (see Wishart, 1993, 1996).

There were, however, important qualitative differences in how the children approached each of these four tasks at different stages in their development. There were also related differences in the timing and nature of child-led social interactions during task presentation. Very often, despite first success being achieved at an encouraging age, performance thereafter proved to be unstable on tasks. These failures in later sessions on tasks which should have been developmentally 'easy' were sometimes the result of a refusal to engage in sufficient trials to be credited with a pass (4/4), not the consequence of any clearly erroneous search on any trial. Success could sometimes be restored by hiding chocolate or a rusk instead of a toy but this strategy was not always successful. More typically, although watching the hiding sequence carefully and clearly capable of precise search, the children would simply either sweep both cups to the floor or pick the same cup on each trial, a very low-level strategy which at best would give a 50 per cent return rate (and, of course, scored as a 'fail').

Low-level engagement with developmentally 'easy' tasks was not the only problem evidenced. Counter-productive behaviours were also frequently produced in response to tasks which were 'difficult', that is, in terms of a given infant's current developmental level. In this case, engagement was much more unambiguously withdrawn, with difficult tasks often actively avoided after only one or two trials, either with protests or simply by resorting to diversionary strategies – such as pretending to be very interested in something else, producing some sort of 'party-trick' to divert the tester into off-task activity, or simply turning on the charm. It is striking how well these behaviours match the social stereotype of Down syndrome – but they were being produced at very specific times, when things were getting difficult for the child. All of the behaviours produced were ones commonly seen in typically developing infants, but these ill-timed social ploys stood out like a sore thumb, with the difference lying in the use to which they were being put. Control children were also sociable and initiated social interactions with the tester but they tended to restrict this to between trials. They also typically worked hard at all levels of the tasks, regardless of whether these were above or below their current developmental level in terms of difficulty. Losses of attention were usually short and re-engagement seldom difficult to obtain. Typically developing children seem to enjoy showing off their abilities and we need to wonder why it is that children with Down syndrome would rather respond in a way that avoids running the risk of error, even in situations where success might well be within their grasp.

The instability in performance seen in our studies suggests a need for great caution if attempting to assess current developmental stage in any child with Down syndrome. If early skills are poorly consolidated and if task engagement is sometimes far from optimal, it would be easy to conclude mistakenly that a child has not yet reached a particular stage in development when in fact they might well be able to succeed on tasks which are developmentally more difficult. In research on children with Down syndrome and in assessing children with Down syndrome, we make great use of psychometric tests, tests that have been standardized on typically developing children – the Bayley Scales of Infant Development, the Stanford Binet Test, or the Wechsler Scales of Intelligence, for instance. The validity of such tests rests on the assumption that test performance will be a reasonably accurate reflection of the skills available to the child and that all children will be equally motivated to demonstrate those skills in a test setting. This seems a very risky assumption in the case of young children with Down syndrome.

The findings reported here suggest that as experience of learning grows, children with Down syndrome may evolve a range of subtle (and sometimes not so subtle) strategies to 'opt out' of learning opportunities. Even when willing to engage in problem-solving tasks, less than efficient use is frequently made of existing cognitive skills. When new skills are eventually acquired, these are all too often inadequately consolidated. An increasing reluctance to take the initiative in learning becomes evident as the children grow older and many seem prepared to wait for learning opportunities to come to them rather than to actively explore the world around them (Wishart, 1991). As the children's partners in learning, it is important that we are alert to these patterns and do not unwittingly collude in their attempts to avoid the cognitive challenges which are central to achieving a working understanding of the physical and social world in which we all live.

References

Avramidis E, Bayliss P, Burden R (2000) A survey into mainstream teachers' attitudes towards the inclusion of children with special educational needs in the ordinary school in one local education authority. Educational Psychology 20: 191–211.

Baird PA, Sadovnik AD (1988) Life expectancy in Down syndrome adults. Lancet: 1354–6.

Carr J (1995) Down's Syndrome: Children Growing Up. Cambridge: Cambridge University Press.

Cicchetti D, Beeghly M (Eds) (1990) Children with Down's Syndrome: A Developmental Perspective. New York: Cambridge University Press.

Duffy L (1990) The relationship between competence and performance in early development in Down syndrome. Unpublished doctoral dissertation, University of Edinburgh, Scotland.

Forlin C (1995) Educators' beliefs about inclusive practices in Western Australia. British Journal of Special Education 22: 179–85.

Franco F, Wishart JG (1995) The use of pointing and other gestures by young children with Down's syndrome. American Journal on Mental Retardation 100: 160–82.

Stratford B, Gunn P (Eds) (1996) New Approaches to Down Syndrome. London: Cassell.

Wishart JG (1987) Performance of 3-5 year old Down's syndrome and non-handicapped children on Piagetian infant search tasks. American Journal of Mental Deficiency 92: 169–77.

Wishart JG (1991) Taking the initiative in learning: a developmental investigation of infants with Down's syndrome. International Journal of Disability, Development and Education 38: 27–44.

Wishart JG (1993) The development of learning difficulties in children with Down's syndrome. Journal of Intellectual Disability Research 37: 389–403.

Wishart JG (1996) Avoidant learning styles and cognitive development in young children with Down syndrome. In Stratford B, Gunn P (Eds) New Approaches to Down Syndrome. London: Cassell. pp 173–205.

Wishart JG (1998) Early intervention. In Fraser WI, Sines D, Kerr M (Eds) Hallas: The Care of People with Intellectual Disabilities (9th ed). Oxford: Butterworth Heinemann. pp 26–35.

Wishart JG, Duffy L (1990) Instability of performance on cognitive tests in infants and young children with Down's syndrome. British Journal of Educational Psychology 59: 10–22.

Wishart JG, Johnston F (1990) The effects of experience on attribution of a stereotyped personality to children with Down's syndrome. Journal of Mental Deficiency Research 34: 409–20.

Wishart JG, Manning G (1996) Trainee teachers' attitudes to inclusive education for children with Down's syndrome. Journal of Intellectual Disability Research 40: 56–65.

CHAPTER 3
Self-regulation in children and young people with Down syndrome

SHEILA GLENN AND CLIFF CUNNINGHAM

Self-regulation has been regarded as one of the key features of development in both typically developing children and children with Down syndrome (Cuskelly, Zhang and Gilmore, 1998). Whitman (1990) even postulated that intellectual disability could best be described as a self-regulatory disorder. Others have emphasized its importance in the process of socialization of children (e.g. Kopp, 1982), and in self-assertion, the capacity to exercise choice and initiate and regulate activities (e.g. Bandura, 1997). Both these perspectives note the importance of attentional mechanisms, which are also highlighted by the difficulties experienced by children with attentional deficit disorder, or hyperactivity, who fail to regulate their behaviour in a socially acceptable way. The antecedents of self-regulation can be seen from birth. For example, in the first weeks of life, infants can regulate levels of social stimulation, and hence their state, through the use of eye gaze and social responses (e.g. Brazelton, 1973). Behavioural strategies for emotion regulation are also seen throughout the first 12 months of life in, for example, self-comforting, help seeking, and avoidance behaviours (e.g. Kopp, 1982). In addition to these inherent propensities, all perspectives highlight the role of the caregiving environment in helping the child to develop self-regulation.

Self-regulation has also been seen as part of a wider conceptualization of the self. The self is usually divided into, first, what someone knows about self, i.e. self-concept; second, what someone feels about self, i.e. self-esteem, which involves understanding self and comparing self to others, together with feelings of self-efficacy. The third component is self-regulation (sometimes studied as autonomy, self-determination, independence, compliance, self-control). This in turn is linked to the development of conscience, and hence moral development (Houch and Spegman, 1999).

Self-regulation, therefore, is a multi-faceted concept. Two theoretical strands can be distinguished which have influenced the empirical studies

28

described in this chapter. The first focuses on theories which emphasize the development of autonomy, initiative and self-efficacy (e.g. Bandura, 1997), and the second on those which emphasize self-control and the need to be aware of situational social demands (e.g. Mischel and Mischel, 1983). Neither of these has received much attention in Down syndrome. In this chapter the first study described is on mastery motivation in infants with Down syndrome, and the second is a study of private speech in young adults with Down syndrome. The final section will try to bring together these somewhat disparate findings, and consider implications for practice and research.

I: Mastery motivation

Mastery motivation has been defined as an intrinsic motivational force to achieve and improve skills, and to master the environment. White (1959) proposed that children have an urge towards competence; they want to have an effect on their environment, and this is shown in their self-directed exploratory and play behaviour. Harter referred to the 'desire to solve cognitively challenging problems for gratification inherent in discovering the solution' (1975: 370). For young children with developmental delays, reports suggest that this intrinsic motivation is lowered (e.g. Harter and Zigler, 1974). There is a lack of consensus as to whether such children are intrinsically lower in motivation because of lower intelligence, as proposed by Sternberg (1985), or whether their lower levels are due to repeated adverse environmental experiences (e.g. Brinker and Lewis, 1982; Diener and Dweck, 1978). Brinker and Lewis (1982), for example, highlighted the problems faced by infants with severe learning difficulties in perceiving that they could affect their environments. They argued that the infants had fewer opportunities to develop such awareness not only due to deficits in sensory, motor and/or memory abilities, but also because caregivers had low expectations and consequently different ways of working with the child. The result is likely to be decreased motivation. With school age children, Diener and Dweck (1978) showed that repeated failure experiences lowered children's motivation to tackle tasks. For children with Down syndrome, Cicchetti and Ganiban (1990) argued that an additional factor is that motivation is diminished due to low arousal levels.

There has been relatively little research on mastery motivation in infants with Down syndrome. MacTurk et al. (1985) studied 11 infants with Down syndrome matched for mental age with 6-month-old typically developing infants. No differences in amounts of goal-directed or off-task behaviour were found. They did however find more looking in infants with Down syndrome and less simple exploration and social behaviour. They concluded that the two groups were equally motivated, but differed in how their motivation was directed. Ruskin, Mundy, Kasari and Sigman (1994a) assessed 42 infants with Down syndrome with 26 mental age (MA) matched typically developing infants (mean MA: 17 months). Using both cause-and-effect and shape-sorting tasks, they also found no differences in level of mastery, with both groups showing higher-level mastery with the cause-and-effect toys. Although no children with Down syndrome were included, Hauser-Cram (1996) similarly reported no differences in mastery motivation at 18 months MA for 25 infants with motor impairments, 25 infants with developmental delay, and 25 typically developing infants. Again she found more motivation on a cause-and-effect task. Previously she reported a similar result for cause-and-effect toys for 34 infants with Down syndrome of 17 months MA (Hauser-Cram, 1993). All these results, although at different MAs, suggest that, in the early years, infants with Down syndrome and others show similar amounts of mastery motivation at similar developmental levels. There is, however, some suggestion that they may distribute motivation differently.

Another question addressed is which environmental factors may affect mastery motivation in Down syndrome. Lewis and Goldberg (1969) argued that a key influence in mastery motivation is the perception of one's self as being effective. This comes about because the environment is responsive to the child's actions; in the early months of life this is dependent on caregivers' sensitive and responsive interactions with the child. There have been several reports of greater maternal directiveness and control in interactions with their infants with Down syndrome (e.g. Crawley and Spiker, 1983; Mahoney and Robenhalt, 1985; Tannock, 1988). Interpretations of this finding have differed. Some (e.g. Berger, 1990) see this greater directiveness as detrimental to the infant's development; others (e.g. Tannock, 1988) argue that directiveness has an important support function, as it enables children with Down syndrome to participate more fully in interactions. In relation to older children with Down syndrome, researchers have speculated that the highly structured programmes often implemented for such children, may actually work to reduce intrinsic motivation (e.g. Cunningham and Glenn, 1985). Jobling (1996) also argued that these tasks may divert children's attention away from the task itself, and more towards social partners. This notion is compatible with the results of a study by Ruskin et al. (1994b). They assessed the social mastery of infants (mean MA: 17 months) during face-to-face play with the researcher. Compared with typically developing infants, they found that infants with Down syndrome were more focused, less likely to show off-task behaviour, and more likely to join in singing. This could possibly be due to infants with Down syndrome having more motivation towards social than object mastery, perhaps because of negative experiences with objects. Alternatively it could be that more input from another person is necessary due to lack of intrinsic control. In one of the few studies with parents, Hauser-Cram (1993) researched 34 infants with Down syndrome who were 3 years of age (mean MA: 19 months), and found that parents who provided appropriate toys and games had children who later showed more persistence. High levels of structure and encouragement were significantly correlated with low levels of independent mastery behaviour in the children.

As reported above, there is little evidence for less mastery behaviour in infants with Down syndrome. However, because studies of this behaviour have been cross-sectional, they have not addressed the issue of how mastery behaviour develops over time. In order to explore this further we used a quasi-longitudinal design. We assessed mastery behaviour in 15 infants with Down syndrome at 6 and 12 months, 15 infants at 12 and 18 months, and 15 infants at 18 and 24 months developmental age (i.e. a total sample of 45). They were matched for MA with 20 typically developing children who were assessed at 6, 12, 18 and 24 months MA (Dayus, 1999; Dayus, Glenn and Cunningham, in preparation). Structured mastery motivation tasks (Morgan, Busch-Rossnagel, Maslin-Cole and Harmon, 1992a) were used; the researcher demonstrated the task to the child, who was then encouraged to attempt it without assistance. The child's behaviour was rated for task directedness, task pleasure and task persistence based on the Morgan et al. (1992a) indices of mastery. Tasks were chosen to be challenging, i.e. neither too easy, nor too difficult, for each individual child. Parent–infant interaction was explored using a different challenging toy. Parental behaviour was rated for activity, dominance/directiveness, encouragement/ assistance and responsivity. Finally parents were asked to rate the child's mastery behaviour using the Dimensions of Mastery Questionnaire (DMQ: Morgan et al., 1992b).

As predicted from the previous studies there were no differences in total mastery behaviours at 6, 18 and 24 months. Mastery behaviours were significantly different at 12 months of age, when the typically developing children showed more mastery on all measures than those with Down syndrome. This appeared to be due to delay in development because the typically developing children significantly increased their mastery behaviours between 6 and 12 months, and the infants with Down syndrome showed the same increase between 12 and 18 months.

As seen in previous studies, the infants with Down syndrome showed significantly more mastery behaviour with cause-and-effect toys than other toys at 6, 12 and 18 months. At 24 months, however, they began to be more motivated by puzzles. In the typically developing children cause-and-effect toys produced more mastery behaviour at 12 months but less at 18 and 24 months. Thus both groups do show a similar pattern. The question arises as to the difference between these tasks. The cause-and-effect toys tend to provide immediate feedback, whereas puzzles require a series of actions to complete a task; thus an end goal has to be kept in mind, and an ability to integrate part/whole relations is required. It may be that by 18 months the typically developing children were shifting from sensorimotor to symbolic functioning, had developed the ability to think in terms of end goals, and therefore found the cause-and-effect toys less challenging. This did not occur until 24 months for the children with Down syndrome, and again suggests a developmental lag for these children. Some support for this was recently provided by Vlachou and Farrell (2000), who found that older children with Down syndrome (mean MA: 3 years, 6 months) showed less mastery with effect-production than problem-solving tasks. Caution is necessary in the interpretation of their results because of methodological problems which include a sample of only four children with Down syndrome, and toys that were not chosen to be challenging for individual children.

In contrast to the structured assessments of mastery, the parents of the children with Down syndrome rated them as less motivated than the parents of the typically developing children at all four assessment ages. It may be that these parents of infants with Down syndrome were comparing them with children of the same chronological age rather than developmental level. Whatever the reason, this judgement was also reflected in the behaviour of parents when interacting with their infants. Overall, mothers of infants with Down syndrome were significantly more dominant and directive than those of the typically developing infants, at all ages tested. Again this confirms previous work.

When maternal interactive style was related to mastery behaviour, there was only one significant correlation at 12 months for the typically developing group: task pleasure was negatively correlated with maternal dominance. For the group with Down syndrome, however, there were significant relationships at all ages. Mastery behaviour in the children was negatively associated with high activity, dominance and directiveness from mothers, and positively associated with encouragement and assistance. Gilmore (2000) studied older infants with Down syndrome, ranging from 24 to 36 months MA, and found similar results. Observed maternal support for autonomy (i.e. the extent to which a mother encourages her child's independent attempts at a task) was significantly related to mastery behaviours only for the children with Down syndrome. She also found no significant group differences in mastery motivation assessed on structured tasks and that the mothers of children with Down syndrome rated their children's persistence as lower than that of the typically developing children.

The causal direction of these associations is not clear. Does highly directive behaviour produce children with low levels of mastery behaviour? Or do parents have to try harder with less aroused children, i.e. do parents try to 'wind them up'? Is it easier to encourage children who show independent behaviour? An intervention study by Seifer, Clark and Sameroff (1991) used interaction coaching and found a positive effect on infant development. To our knowledge there are no intervention studies using mastery behaviour as an outcome measure, which is necessary to address these issues.

Within the constraints of this evidence, one can conclude that low mastery motivation is not inevitable in Down syndrome. Its pattern and direction may be different and delayed because of their maturational delay and cognitive difficulties. They do appear to require more 'external regulation' from sensitive caregivers than typically developing infants. But they still need and respond to the intrinsic motivation of challenge.

II: Private speech

Speech directed to self and to no particular listener (private speech) is regarded as critically important for self-regulation (Whitman, 1990; Vygotsky, 1962). It is very common in children's development: Berk (1994) recently estimated that private speech accounts for 20 to 60 per cent of the speech of children less than ten years old. As children grow older private speech becomes covert, is no longer audible to a listener, but retains its self-regulating function.

Mead (1934) proposed a hierarchy of development from pre-social self-stimulatory word play, leading to outward-directed private speech (to objects as well as to others and self), and then to inward-directed private speech or dialogue with self. This eventually changes to inaudible muttering, and finally to silent inner speech. Central to Mead's argument was that the different types of private speech were all functionally related to the development of the concept of self. As the concept of self develops children are able to have a dialogue with themselves, develop chains of thought, and hence be self-directing.

Vygotsky (1962) similarly believed that private speech was communication with self for the purpose of guiding one's own thought processes and actions. He also argued that make-believe and fantasy are particularly important in development, as they allow children to set their own challenges, goals and actions towards those goals. In this sense it is like free play, in that external controls and demands, which may inhibit the behaviour, are absent. He noted that every episode of make-believe requires children to create imaginary situations where they follow social rules. For example, a child imagining herself to be a mother and a doll to be a child is following the rules of parent and child behaviour. His view is supported by evidence of the frequency of private speech in fantasy play situations (e.g. Krafft and Berk, 1998).

Turning to children with Down syndrome, one might expect them to have difficulties with self-regulation through private speech, due to the problem with expressive language seen in this syndrome. However, no work on this aspect of private speech was found in the literature. The limited literature found largely referred to observations on older children and adults talking out loud to themselves, and related this to social isolation (possibly due to communication difficulties), and/or emotional/psychiatric disorders, and/or behaviour problems (Buckley and Sacks, 1987; Shepperdson, 1992; Fotheringham and Thompson, 1994). When we began a study on transition to adult life and self-concept with 77 young people with Down syndrome and their families in the Manchester Down Syndrome Cohort (Cunningham, 1996), many parents reported that their young adult with Down syndrome talked out loud to themselves or to objects, and some expressed concern. In an extreme instance the young person was seen by a therapist and given medication in an attempt to stop this behaviour. Thus private speech appeared to be interpreted mainly from a pathological perspective. An alternative hypothesis was that private speech is common and follows Mead's developmental model. Since the developmental level of most young people with Down syndrome is less than ten years (Cunningham, 1988; Carr, 1995), private speech could be viewed as developmentally appropriate and, within a Vygotskyan framework, important for self-regulation; it has not yet become internalized as silent inner speech.

To explore this further, the parents of the young adults with Down syndrome were asked whether or not the young person talked out loud to themselves, where this talk occurred, and what they talked about. Their responses were related to the young person's verbal mental age (VMA), measured on the British Picture Vocabulary Scale to provide an approximation of developmental level; to communication skills rated from observations during interviews with the young person; to the amount of their social contacts; and to any behavioural difficulties, rated from interviews with parents. The method is detailed in Glenn and Cunningham (2000). Results showed that the vast majority of these young people (91 per cent) either talked to themselves currently (86 per cent) or had done so in the past (5 per cent). The latter had the highest VMA, whereas those who had never used private speech were below the 15th percentile of VMA for this group. Those who only used private speech when alone in their rooms had significantly higher VMAs than those who used private speech in front of others. The latter may have not yet learned the social rule that talking out loud to self is not considered as appropriate in front of others. Clearly they were different in terms of their self-regulatory social behaviour, but they were not different in social contact scores or in communication abilities. Thus there was no support for the view that private speech arises because of social isolation or communication problems. One caveat is that most of this sample had full social lives, and one parent felt that the incidence of private speech in her daughter had increased as her social contacts had decreased.

Fifty-three parents were able to describe the content of private speech. Seventy per cent was self dialogue involving either fantasy – for example:

> . . . she has an imagination beyond belief. You can hear her talking in her room. Working for a big boss, singing, being on TV, getting paid. Often hear her talking with characters from the soaps;

or going over recent events or future plans:

> Always has since she was a little girl . . . still does this talk to self about events or what she will do.

Thirteen per cent was talk to objects (for example, talking to a cassette player – 'Are you going to sleep? Hurry up'), and 15 per cent self-direction (for example – 'She'll give herself instructions about what to wear'). Those involved in fantasy (which included those with imaginary friends) had slightly higher VMAs and communication abilities than those going over real life events. Thus, again, there was no suggestion that they were particularly poor communicators, or that they were more socially isolated. Taylor (1999) similarly found with typically developing children that those with imaginary friends often displayed advanced social understanding; they were not, as often feared by parents, loners. The present study also found that the young people who engaged in fantasy private speech had lower rates of behavioural difficulties than the average for the total sample.

It would appear that these young people with Down syndrome use private speech in the same way as expected of younger people of equivalent developmental levels. This suggests that the functions are the same, viz: self-communication for self-regulation and the practice of social competence. Difficulties arise for parents because this private speech is not age-appropriate; adults are not expected to talk out loud to themselves, and it is typically interpreted as indicating pathology. However, rather than trying to suppress a behaviour which seems critically important for self-regulation, parents might be advised to help the young person to discriminate settings where it is and is not appropriate, which in itself is enhancing their self-regulatory behaviour. If there are worrying changes in behaviour including private speech, then this may be symptomatic of some mental stress. In such an instance, it would be more important to tackle the underlying cause, rather than trying to get rid of the private speech.

Implications for practice and further research

These two very different studies of individuals with Down syndrome have demonstrated that self-regulatory behaviours are present in both infancy and young adulthood, and that these behaviours are much as one would expect from models of typical development. There is evidence for developmental delay, i.e. the development of individuals with Down syndrome follows the same pattern as other people but the rate is slower and there are more extensive plateaux of little measurable developmental progress. But this is expected as it is found in most other areas, e.g. linguistic, motor, and cognitive growth. Both studies also give some indication that environmental factors can influence self-regulatory behaviour.

For mastery motivation, we found that parents of infants with Down syndrome were more directive and seemed to try harder to provoke a response. This is expected from present literature. It may be that they viewed the session of being observed playing with the child as a test and so tried harder to demonstrate their child's abilities. If this is the case they may interact less directively in 'non-test' situations. More extensive observational studies of natural behaviour in a home setting would be needed to investigate this issue. The infants with Down syndrome whose mothers were more highly directive showed fewer independent mastery behaviours. This is again indicated in previous literature. What is not known is whether the major influence comes from the mother or the child. Is the mother provoked to more directiveness and activity in face of the child's apparent low arousal and initiative, or is the behaviour based on a belief that this is how one best helps 'these' children? We suspect that both partners are influential, but an intervention study is required to answer this question. In the absence of this we would advise parents that they may need to be more directive of interactions in order to gain the child's attention and interest. However, they need to be sensitive and responsive to the child's cues and withdraw support/control when the child is trying to explore and work independently. They should also reward and encourage self-regulatory behaviours when any opportunity occurs.

Private speech should be seen as an adaptive functional behaviour, which should not be discouraged. However as the child gets older he or she needs to learn the social rules and that talking out loud to self is not socially acceptable. Learning this is a self-regulatory behaviour, just as private speech is self-regulatory. What we do not know is whether one can teach older people with Down syndrome to control their speaking out loud when they are at the developmental level at which it is very common. In other words, is the natural drive for private speech greater than the ability to inhibit it; does the ability to inhibit it depend on cognitive development? Again, one needs to set up intervention studies to teach older children with Down syndrome who speak out loud how to self-regulate the behaviour.

These two disparate and exploratory studies have just touched the surface of the multi-faceted area called self-regulation. They highlight the importance of further study of these two areas and more extensive exploration of self-regulatory behaviours in children and adults with Down syndrome. We believe the area is of equal or greater importance than many aspects of the current curriculum.

References

Bandura A (1997) Self-efficacy: The Exercise of Control. New York: W.H. Freeman and Company.

Berger J (1990) Interactions between parents and their infants with Down syndrome. In Cicchetti D, Beeghly M (Eds) Children with Down Syndrome: A Developmental Perspective. New York: Cambridge University Press. pp 101-46.

Berk LE (1994) Why children talk to themselves. Scientific American 271(November): 60-5.

Brazelton TB (1973) Neonatal Behavioral Assessment Scale. Philadelphia: J.B. Lippincott.

Brinker RP, Lewis M (1982) Discovering the competent handicapped infant: a process approach to assessment and intervention. Topics in Early Childhood Education 2: 1-16.

Buckley S, Sacks B (1987). The Adolescent with Down's Syndrome. Portsmouth: Down's Syndrome Trust.

Carr J (1995) Down's Syndrome: Children Growing Up. Cambridge: Cambridge University Press.

Cicchetti D, Ganiban J (1990) The organization and coherence of developmental processes in infants and children with Down syndrome. In Hodapp RM, Burack JA, Zigler E (Eds) Issues in the Developmental Approach to Mental Retardation. New York: Cambridge University Press.

Crawley SB, Spiker D (1983) Mother-child interactions involving two-year-olds with Down syndrome: a look at individual differences. Child Development 54: 1312-23.

Cunningham CC (1988) Down's Syndrome: An Introduction for Parents. London: Souvenir Press.

Cunningham CC (1996) Families of children with Down syndrome. Down Syndrome: Research and Practice 4: 87-95.

Cunningham CC, Glenn SM (1985) Parental involvement and early intervention. In Stratford B, Lane D (Eds) Current Approaches to Down Syndrome. London: Holt, Rinehart and Winston. pp 347-62.

Cuskelly M, Zhang A, Gilmore L (1998) The importance of self-regulation in young children with Down syndrome. International Journal of Disability, Development and Education 45: 331-41.

Dayus B (1999) The development of mastery motivation in infants with Down syndrome. Unpublished PhD thesis, John Moores University, Liverpool, UK.

Dayus B, Glenn SM, Cunningham CC (in preparation) The development of mastery motivation in infants with Down syndrome. Available from S. Glenn.

Diener CI, Dweck CS (1978) An analysis of learned helplessness II: The processing of success. Journal of Personality and Social Psychology 39: 940-53.

Fotheringham JB, Thompson F (1994) Case-report of a person with Down's syndrome and multiple personality-disorder. Canadian Journal of Psychiatry 39: 116-19.

Gilmore L (2000) Mastery motivation, self-regulation and maternal support for autonomy: a comparative study of young children with Down syndrome. Unpublished PhD thesis, University of Queensland, Brisbane, Australia.

Glenn SM, Cunningham CC (2000) Parents' reports of young people with Down syndrome talking out loud to themselves. Mental Retardation 38: 498-505.

Harter S (1975) Developmental differences in the manifestation of mastery motivation on problem-solving tasks. Child Development 46: 370-8.

Harter S, Zigler E (1974) The assessment of effectance motivation in normal and retarded children. Developmental Psychology 10: 169-80.

Hauser-Cram P (1993) Mastery motivation in three-year-old children with Down syndrome. In Messer D (Ed) Mastery Motivation in Early Childhood: Development, Measurement and Social Processes. London: Routledge. pp 230-50.

Hauser-Cram P (1996) Mastery motivation in toddlers with developmental disabilities. Child Development 67: 236-48.

Houch GM, Spegman AM (1999) The development of self: theoretical understandings and conceptual underpinnings. Infants and Young Children 12: 1-16.

Jobling A (1996) Play. In Stratford B, Gunn P (Eds) New Approaches to Down Syndrome. London: Cassell. pp 379-401.

Kopp C (1982) Antecedents of self-regulation: a developmental perspective. Developmental Psychology 18: 199-214.

Krafft KC, Berk LE (1998) Private speech in two pre-schools: significance of open-ended activities and make-believe play for verbal self-regulation. Early Childhood Research Quarterly 13: 637-58.

Lewis M, Goldberg S (1969) Perceptual-cognitive development in infancy: a generalized expectancy model as a function of the mother-infant interaction. Merrill-Palmer Quarterly 15: 81-100.

MacTurk R, Vietze P, McCarthy M, McQuiston S, Yarrow L (1985) The organization of exploratory behavior in Down syndrome and non-delayed infants. Child Development 56: 573-87.

Mahoney G, Robenhalt K (1985) A comparison of conversational patterns between mothers and their Down syndrome and normal infants. Journal of the Division of Early Childhood 10: 172-80.

Mead GH (1934). Mind, Self and Society. Chicago: University of Chicago Press.

Mischel W, Mischel HN (1983) Development of children's knowledge of self-control strategies. Child Development 54: 603-19.

Morgan GA, Busch-Rossnagel NA, Maslin-Cole CA, Harmon RJ (1992a) Mastery Motivation Tasks: Manual for 15- to 36-month-old Children. The Bronx: Fordham University, Psychology Department.

Morgan GA, Maslin-Cole CA, Harmon RJ, Busch-Rossnagel NA, Jennings KD, Hauser-Cram P, Brockman LM (1992b) Assessing Perceptions of Mastery Motivation: The Dimensions of Mastery Questionnaire, its Development, Psychometrics and Use. Colorado State University, Human Development and Family Studies Department.

Ruskin EM, Mundy P, Kasari C, Sigman M (1994a) Object mastery motivation of children with Down syndrome. American Journal on Mental Retardation 98: 499-509.

Ruskin EM, Mundy P, Kasari C, Sigman M (1994b) Attention to people and toys during social and object mastery in children with Down syndrome. American Journal on Mental Retardation 99: 103-11.

Seifer R, Clark GN, Sameroff AJ (1991) Positive effects of interaction coaching on infants with developmental disabilities and their mothers. American Journal on Mental Retardation 96: 1–11.

Shepperdson B (1992). A longitudinal study of a cohort of people with Down's Syndrome. Final report to ESRC, Swindon, UK.

Sternberg RJ (1985) Beyond IQ: A Triarchic Theory of Human Intelligence. New York: Cambridge University Press.

Tannock R (1988) Mothers' directiveness in their interactions with their children with and without Down syndrome. American Journal on Mental Retardation 93: 154–65.

Taylor M (1999) Imaginary Companions and the Children who Create Them. Oxford: Oxford University Press.

Vlachou M, Farrell P (2000) Object mastery motivation in pre-school children with and without disabilities. Educational Psychology 20: 167–76.

Vygotsky L (1962) Thought and Language. Cambridge, MA: MIT Press.

White RW (1959) Motivation reconsidered: the concept of competence. Psychological Review 66: 297–333.

Whitman TL (1990) Self-regulation and mental retardation. American Journal on Mental Retardation 94: 347–62.

SECTION 3
EDUCATIONAL PROVISION

Introduction

Early intervention has become an accepted part of the educational provision for young children with disabilities in most western countries. Both its form and its focus have changed over the years since education for very young children was first introduced and Robin Treloar and Sue Cairns' chapter reviewing the changes that occurred in the provision of this type of service in Australia helps us understand the bases for these shifts. Their paper is not just an historical account however but makes a clear statement of their views about what is required for effective services in the early years.

The authors chose to focus on several central elements of early intervention which they see as having changed over the 25 years. They suggest that research has led a change in the way early intervention is conceived (family-focused rather than purely child-focused), and the way interventions are conducted (play-based rather than direct instruction). Language learning is used as an example of the move to more naturalistic intervention methods, which the authors argue are important if children are to continue to be engaged with the learning process. Connections to the earlier section on motivation can be readily seen.

Loretta Giorcelli has written a challenging paper about educational provision for children with special needs. She argues that regular educational environments are not yet as good as they could be in meeting the academic needs of children with disabilities. Her chapter has two main thrusts: (1) we need to keep improving our services to students with special needs through a proper recognition of the barriers that currently prevent the delivery of a completely effective education; and (2) we need to continue to examine our assumptions about what comprises an appropriate educational delivery system for students with special learning needs.

In addition to raising some issues that will require continued research and discussion before they are resolved, Giorcelli also provides some quite specific advice to schools and teachers about strategies which have already been shown to improve the schooling experience of children with special needs.

40

CHAPTER 4
What matters most? A reflection on a quarter century of early childhood intervention

ROBIN TRELOAR AND SUSAN CAIRNS

This paper is essentially a reflection – it presents our practitioners' perspective, within an Australian context. We acknowledge the limitations of this perspective, both in relation to that of parents of children with disabilities, and in relation to diverse cultural contexts in which the readers of this paper live and work.

The writers of this paper are special educators who began their careers in the Macquarie University Down Syndrome Program in Sydney, Australia, in the mid- to late-1970s. The Macquarie Program was one of Australia's first early intervention programs for children with intellectual disabilities, and it had a powerful impact on the development of services, through dissemination of information, research, teacher training and curriculum development. Some 25 years on from the beginnings of the Macquarie Program, we find ourselves looking forwards into the new century with some concerns. How can we make limited resources meet the increasing demands on our services? Are we doing things in the best possible way? Why do we do things this way? What does the process of change over the past 25 years tell us about why we do what we do?

We begin with a brief look back at the early years of the Macquarie Program, partly because of the writers' personal involvement in the program, but also because it represents a starting point for this discussion of change.

In 1974, Moira Pieterse began seeing mothers and their babies with Down syndrome in her office. Those mothers and babies were there because of a response to a set of new ideas which together seemed to offer a radical new perspective on the potential of people with intellectual disabilities. To simplify, these influences were:

- New techniques in special education – mainly behavioural techniques – which were demonstrably enabling school aged children with intellectual disabilities to learn;

41

- New thinking about mother–baby bonding, and research by Trevarthen and others which showed how a mother's interaction patterns influence the behaviour patterns of her infant (see, for example, Trevarthen and Hubley, 1978);
- The beginnings of reports coming out of Seattle, Washington, suggesting that young children with Down syndrome could respond to educational intervention (see, for example, Hayden and Dmitriev, 1975).

What did the Macquarie Program, and similar programs developing throughout the world, offer in those early years?

Optimism, hope, positive expectations

At this time, children with Down syndrome were classified as trainable in matters such as basic self-help skills, but as non-educable. At Macquarie, the message was 'Let's not limit children by our negative expectations'.

An educational model

The focus was not on *treating* children, but on teaching them. Even the therapy staff became teachers – teaching the parents, certainly, but also teaching the children skills in movement and balance, through the building of confidence and enjoyment. Part of the educational model was a *curriculum* based on a fine breakdown of the steps of normal early childhood development. There was also a strong emphasis on the use of *effective teaching strategies,* in both structured and play-based contexts, and on measuring outcomes.

A family-focused model

Our thinking about how to work with families has shifted over recent years. We look back at some of our own practices in working with families with the recognition that there were times when, instead of providing support, we caused additional stress. Nevertheless, the Macquarie Program, and other early programs like it, gave credit to the power of families, and the resourcefulness of families, in a way that was quite new.

A focus on integration

The Macquarie Program was committed to integration in the community, in regular early childhood settings, and most radically of all, in regular schools. We believed with a passion that children with Down syndrome had a right to the opportunities and experiences available to all children in the community. We backed this up with support and training for teachers. It was a concept that was embraced warily, but often warmly, by those mainstream educators who agreed to get involved. For them, for us, and for many of the families, there was a sense of being part of something that was new, exciting and inherently right. There was a sense of mission.

We have chosen to look at some of the key changes in the practice of early intervention over the years in terms of three themes: research, the challenges of growth and change, and conceptual shifts.

Research

Of course, thinking began to evolve and change immediately following the introduction of early intervention programmes, and the earliest influence on thinking, and a continuing key influence, was research. It is beyond the scope of this chapter to do any justice to research-based changes in practice – instead we will touch briefly on just two areas.

Research in language development

The Macquarie Program began to teach children to understand language and to talk using a behavioural approach that utilized controlled cues and reinforcement, a carefully sequenced curriculum and rigorous documentation of what children actually did and said. At the same time, there was focus on reciprocal parent–infant interactions: a focus which valued interactions in natural environments during all the shared activities of the day. It became increasingly evident that these interactions were valuable not only in strengthening the bond between parent and child, and increasing the child's general responsiveness, but also in extending the child's expressive and receptive language skills.

Amongst the many publications which reinforced this concept, the Macquarie staff were particularly influenced by one by McLean and Snyder-McLean: *A Transactional Approach to Early Language Training* (1978). This work helped us to understand not only the theoretical basis for teaching language in natural settings, but ways in which we might operationalize this theory. A series of strategies evolved – in parallel to similar developments all over the world in response to the new research – which were embedded within play and daily routines and could be implemented by all adults involved with the child. Taking turns, following the child's lead, matching the model to the child's interest, waiting for a response, minimizing directions, attending to content and intention over form, using conversational responses both to affirm and extend – all these critical strategies, and more, evolved at this time. They have been confirmed and refined in further research, especially in the area of reciprocity (for example, Kaye and Charney, 1980), and have remained integral to our work in language intervention.

Research is continuing to extend our understanding in many areas: for example, the frequency and intensity of reciprocal interactions which correlate with enhanced language development, (Hart and Risley, 1995; Hart, 2000; Mahoney et al., 1998), the relative efficacy of different kinds of elicitation techniques (Yoder, Warren, McCathren and Leew, 1998) and the ways in which we can work with families to develop interventions which are respectful of, and relevant to, the interaction styles and patterns of diverse cultural groups (McCollum and McBride, 1997).

Later studies have greatly refined our understanding of the factors which affect the way in which children with Down syndrome in particular learn to communicate. It was determined quite early that children with Down syndrome had a slower rate of spoken vocabulary development compared with children matched for developmental age (Cardoso-Martins, Mervis and Mervis, 1985). Yet when non-verbal signals are taken into account, we find a significantly higher rate of communication (Franco and Wishart, 1995; Weitzner-Lin, 1997). Gestural communication, like speech, can be affected by muscle tone and coordination difficulties, and can be easy to misinterpret, or miss altogether. In response to such research we have learned to refine our observational skills, and to assist parents and other carers to identify more of the child's communicative attempts. We have been able to refine children's gestures and teach them to use gestural and pictorial symbols.

The results of this are quite profound. Children experience the power of communicating a message earlier than their speech difficulties will allow (Miller, Leddy and Leavitt, 1999). Frustration is averted. Non-intrusive responses to problem behaviours are found. Parents and carers experience more rewarding interactions with their child, which in turn supports their ability to build and maintain reciprocity.

Play-based intervention

A second area in which research has influenced the way we work has been in support for play-based intervention within natural environments. Research gave rise to concerns about generalization from adult-directed, one-to-one instruction, and about the development of dependence on adult cues and prompts (Beckwith, 1976; Mahoney, 1988). In theory, well-planned instruction addressed these concerns, by building in generalization and fading supports.

In practice, these instructional stages could not always be well controlled. If a child with Down syndrome at preschool did not demonstrate curiosity about the environment, or attempt new tasks, or attend to an activity as a member of a group, or persist with challenging activities, was the solution to remove the child for one-to-one instruction, or to work with the child within the environment, increasing his or her engagement, motivation, persever-ance and problem-solving skills? As we moved increasingly towards the latter option, early intervention began to look different.

This shift in the context of instruction carried with it significant challenges. There is certainly a risk that this style of intervention will result in a watering down of effective instruction. 'Follow the child's lead' is sometimes interpreted as 'whatever the child wants to do is fine'. Without the contextual cues of a confined space, prescribed and ordered materials and detailed program sheets, it is easy for adults – including experienced professionals – to lose focus on exactly *why* we are spending this time with this child. In addition to, and very probably as a result of, this challenge, many parents question the efficacy of play-based assessment and place greater value on more formal instruction.

Yet if we implement a play-based approach in a research-based way, we apply it with the same rigour that we applied to adult-directed interven-tions in highly controlled environments (Bricker and Cripe, 1992; Linder, 1983, 1993). The many teachers and therapists with whom we have discussed this issue in preparing this chapter report that they maintain their concern about measurable outcomes for children, and feel just as accountable, or more, when working outside the traditional style and context of their discipline. Our specialist knowledge and understanding of how children learn must be deep-seated if we are to use it flexibly, respond to unplanned opportunities and maintain focus in potentially hectic environments. Play-based intervention demands more complex environ-mental assessment, more time-consuming environmental modifications, and infinitely more sharing among the team of parents and professionals about what works and what does not.

The challenges of growth and social change

Many changes in the field of early childhood intervention relate not so much to the way in which we interact with children, as to the way in which services are delivered. As the concept of early intervention gained accep-tance, and more funding became available, the diversity of families accessing services increased and has continued to increase. Services encountered challenges of how to meet the needs of families from diverse linguistic and cultural backgrounds, with different attitudes to disability and differing child-rearing practices, families in financial difficulties for whom housing and feeding a family was a more pressing need than when their baby rolled or babbled, families in which the parent or parents were affected by post-natal depression, mental illness, intellectual disabilities, family breakdown, domestic violence, substance abuse, and other extreme challenges.

Our concept of what is involved in early intervention had to grow in response to the sheer diversity of families, coupled with a belief that intervention is more effective when it responds to families' individual needs. This has been a key factor in the shift from family-focused services to family-centred services – a shift which we will discuss later in this chapter.

Changing patterns of family life

In Australia, the way in which early intervention services connect with families has had to change not only because of the numbers and diversity of families involved, but also because of widespread social changes over the past quarter century (Hartely, 1995; Gilding, 1997). More families are now isolated from their extended families. Many have little prior knowledge or experience of child rearing, and have limited family support. There is increasing pressure for both parents – or, in the case, of single parent families, the sole carer – to return to work during the child's early years. The cost of childcare means that increasing numbers of children have multiple carers, meaning that more people must become part of the team that builds around each family – more people who need resourcing and training. Fathers are increasingly involved in child rearing, and family-centred principles affirm their role and their rights. Such factors demand greater flexibility in where and when early childhood intervention staff meet with families and what is discussed at these meetings.

Systemic changes

One corollary of growth has been the increasing 'systemization' of early childhood intervention services. In order to cope with increasing pressure on limited resources, agencies within Australia have developed guidelines for eligibility and for access to various service options. Such guidelines are not research driven – there is no clear research to guide us in determining universally effective patterns of frequency or intensity of service.

Such systems reflect a desire to achieve some kind of equity – to be fair to all families. This is valid if we can define 'equity' in terms of inputs, judged on the basis of whether or not families are receiving the same number of visits. If we look at equity in terms of outcomes – whether each family's priorities are being effectively addressed – the picture can look different. Different families have different priorities and needs. The same family may have different needs at different life stages. Do the systems within which we work allow us the opportunity to work in different ways with families in response to their differing needs? This is one of the major challenges we face in planning for the future.

There are, of course, other systemic changes within Australia, and different patterns of change affect different nations. McCollum's (2000) reflection on change in the United States over the course of her career struck some chords. She commented on the impact of the move towards fee-for-service intervention funded by Medicaid or insurance, which appears to be unintentionally bolstering a swing back towards a clinical model of service delivery. She notes that:

> The consequences have been a return to fragmented services at the level of the child and family and less opportunity for collaboration among professionals working with each child and family. It has become much more difficult for service providers of all disciplines to be 'family-centered,' to embed their interventions within the contexts of families' daily lives, and to integrate their interventions with those of other professionals in recognition of the integrated nature of early development.
>
> (McCollum, 2000: 85–6)

The fragmentation that can arise from both agency-based eligibility policy and government approaches to funding illustrates the fragility of the family-centred, integrated, trans-disciplinary model of service delivery which so many have been striving to achieve.

Conceptual shifts

Over the past 25 years there have been some major shifts in the way we think about the service we provide. These shifts have been influenced by research, by social change and also, importantly, by the accumulation of experience. We have alluded above to the profound shifts in our thinking about teamwork: the hard-won alliance between early childhood educators in mainstream services and special educators over the concept of 'developmentally appropriate practice', the evolution of trans-disciplinary teams, and the increasing emphasis on collaborative teamwork – all shifts which have had a significant impact on the way we work. The progression from 'integration' to 'inclusion' – ensuring that children are not only placed, but are active participants in generic early childhood services – has also profoundly influenced the nature and context of early childhood intervention.

But given the necessity to be selective, we feel compelled to give further space to the shift towards family-centred early intervention, a shift which has required professionals to rethink not only how we work, but also what we are in this work to do. The origins of this shift extended beyond early childhood intervention to a broader rethinking, by both social theorists and consumers of social services, of the ways in which families connect to both formal and informal community supports.

Many pioneering early childhood intervention programs, the Macquarie Program among them, began with a family focus, recognizing the importance of the family in supporting and teaching the child and attempting to mobilize this pivotal role to achieve developmental outcomes for the child. In family-centred practice the emphasis is different. Some key tenets which should be evident in the planning process are as follows:

- The diagnosis of a disability does not just happen to a child – it happens to a family.
- Families have a right to control intervention and to make fully informed choices. The relationship between families and professionals is one of *partnership*.
- Intervention focuses on needs and aspirations identified by the family, not by professionals.
- Intervention aims to enhance the family's competence and independence, rather than encouraging dependence.
- Early intervention workers are prepared to engage with families about issues and concerns which are beyond their field of expertise, at least to the point of assisting families to identify appropriate sources of support.

Although not mandated, as in the United States, there is an expectation that every family will have an Individual Family Service Plan, and that this plan will take family concerns and priorities as the starting point. Our own observation is that here in New South Wales, this is not yet happening consistently. What is termed 'family-centred planning' is not always so, in reality, and the gap between research-based best practice and actual practice is a theme of many reflections in the recent literature (see, for example, Bruder, 2000).

The following is a familiar scenario. An 'Individual Family Service Plan' meeting is convened by a case worker, with the aim of developing a plan which clarifies the family's priorities and needs and guides the intervention of everyone involved over the coming months. In this scenario, the case worker invites all those involved with the family – special education teacher, therapists, childcare staff, medical practitioner. The meeting is scheduled during working hours: one parent gets leave from work to come, but the other cannot. At the outset, the case worker says to the parent, 'We are a family-centred service. We're here to find out what is important to you. What are your priorities?' The parent looks around the room full of 'experts' and wonders how to address this huge and complex question. 'You're the experts,' she says, 'Tell us what we should be doing.' Control of the meeting then passes to the professionals, and there is little further reference to the parent, other than to ask, 'Is that OK with you?' It is a brave parent who says, 'No.' Assisting parents to be active participants, and ultimately leaders, in decision-making is a skill which all professionals in the field need continually to hone.

Professionals sometimes express a concern that the family-centred model diminishes the value of professional expertise – that it means doing what parents want even if it is contrary to professional judgement. This is a misrepresentation. For most families, most of the time, the skills and experience of professionals are the main reason that they are involved in early childhood intervention, aside from the support they share with each other. Professional input is more likely to have meaningful outcomes in family-centred services, because it is more likely to be relevant to family priorities and hence more likely to be followed through, day to day. The distinction is that in family-centred services:

- the family's own expertise is also acknowledged and valued; and
- the role of the professional is to assist families to evaluate all options, and to make informed choices, rather than to offer a predetermined 'package'.

It has been observed that it has proved difficult for services to operationalize family-centred practice – to translate the philosophical and theoretical debate into actions and procedures (Bruder, 2000). The New South Wales Ageing and Disability Department (1997) has sponsored the development of recommended practices in family-centred early intervention, a process which has had family input at every stage.

The project outlined many recommended actions and procedures in response to family input (such as that above), the pooling of professional experience and study of the evidence. A brief selection of key practices is as follows:

In first contacts between families and early childhood intervention services, the family member is:

- assured that his or her enquiry is welcome;
- asked for information only when it is needed to answer their enquiry, and given the reasons that such information is being sought;
- actively assisted to locate a service which can help the family, if the agency is unable to do so.

When information is given to families, it is:

- given when the family requests it and repeated as often as the family considers necessary;
- available in different media to suit different needs;
- presented in a way which is respectful of the family's cultural values.

When an assessment of the child is planned, families are:

• fully informed about the options available for carrying out the assessment;
• involved in planning and implementing the assessment;
• given opportunities for immediate discussion, ensuring the family's identified concerns are addressed first.

When developing an Individual Family Service Plan, families are:

• offered choices about the ways in which they want to share information
  about themselves and their child and to participate in the team process;
• offered choices about the location, timing and composition of planning
  meetings;
• given all the preparation and information they need in order to be able to
  participate actively as the key decision-makers for their family.

When working towards a transition to another setting, such as a school,
families are:

• fully informed about the options available to them, and their rights with
  regard to these options;
• given full information about any official requirements (such as assessments or detailed paperwork), and the reasons behind them;
• offered opportunities to link up with other families who are, or have
  recently been, in a similar situation.

In ongoing interactions between early childhood intervention programs and
families, professionals need to:

• monitor the family's ongoing experience of intervention and support
  them as they adjust to changes;
• support the family to attain their stated priorities, respecting each family's
  values, attitudes and culture;
• bring families together to enable them to provide support and share
  expertise with each other.

(Selected from *Recommended Practices in Family-centred Early
Intervention*, New South Wales Ageing and Disability Department, 1997.)

The guidelines from which this small selection is taken reflect the context in
which they were developed: the implication is not that all early childhood

programs, everywhere, should adopt this particular set of guidelines, or any other. The point is that it is not enough for professionals to decide to 'be' family-centred: all of us require concrete, observable, quantifiable descriptors against which to evaluate our practice.

In order to meet their changing needs, families are often required to shift between agencies, and are even sometimes required to transfer altogether to a new and unknown service. It is crucial that we develop more effective ways of working across agencies in support of families, as relationships already established may assist families as they make necessary transitions. We need to take a fresh look at team boundaries – defining teams in terms of partnerships with individual families rather than allegiances to particular agencies. In New South Wales there is some governmental support for effective interagency collaboration, through the Early Childhood Intervention Coordination Program. There is still have a long way to go in ensuring flexibility and informed choice for all families, however, particularly in the face of limited funds and resources.

To conclude this chapter, we would like to offer our own response to the question, 'What matters most?' We are aware that there can be as many responses to this question as there are people to ask it. We are also aware that for many, what matters most will be the means to survive, access to adequate medical care, freedom from discrimination. We are fortunate to be able to approach this question from the relative security of an established tradition of providing early childhood intervention services to families. Hence we offer the following as *some* answers, rather than *the* answers, hoping that they will assist readers to clarify their own responses.

What matters most for a child who has Down Syndrome, or another disability?

- The love and support of a family.
- The care of an inclusive community.
- The opportunity to develop skills which will enrich his or her life and expand his or her choices.

What matters most for a family that has a child with Down syndrome, or another disability?

- The support of other families, within informal networks.
- Responsive, flexible services which respect the family's individuality.
- Support to make fully informed choices on behalf of themselves and their child.

What matters most for us, the writers, as professionals in the field?

- Ongoing input from researchers and fellow practitioners who ask the questions that really matter.
- Flexible systems which support the development of family-friendly work practices, individualized decision making and non-proprietorial attitudes to families.
- Ongoing and open partnerships with the families in whose lives we are privileged to participate.

References

Beckwith L (1976) Caregiver–infant interaction and development of the high-risk infant. In Tjossem T (Ed) Intervention Strategies for High-risk Infants and Young Children. Baltimore: University Park Press. pp 119–39.

Bricker D, Cripe JJW (1992) An Activity-based Approach to Early Intervention. Baltimore: Paul H. Brookes.

Bruder MB (2000) Family-centered early intervention: clarifying our values for the new millennium. Topics in Early Childhood Special Education 20: 105–15.

Cardoso-Martin C, Mervis CV, Mervis CS (1985) Early vocabulary acquisition by children with Down syndrome. American Journal on Mental Deficiency 90: 177–84.

Franco F, Wishart JG (1995) Use of pointing and other gestures by young children with Down syndrome. American Journal on Mental Retardation 100: 160–82.

Gilding M (1997) Australian Families: A Comparative Perspective. Melbourne: Longman.

Hart B (2000) A natural history of early language experience. Topics in Early Childhood Special Education 20: 28–32.

Hart B, Risley T (1995) Meaningful Differences in the Everyday Experiences of Young American Children. Baltimore: Paul H. Brookes.

Hartely R (1995) Families and Cultural Diversity in Australia. Sydney, NSW: Allen and Unwin.

Hayden AH, Dmitriev V (1975) The multidisciplinary preschool programme for Down syndrome children at the University of Washington Model Preschool Centre. In Friedlander BZ, Kirk GE, Sterritt GM (Eds) Exceptional Infant, Vol 3: Assessment and Intervention. New York: Brunner/Mazel.

Kaye K, Charney R (1980) How mothers maintain 'dialogue' with two-year-olds. In Olson DR (Ed) The Social Foundations of Language and Thought: Essays in Honor of Jerome S. Bruner. New York: Norton, 1980. pp 211–30.

Linder TW (1983) Early Childhood Special Education: Program Development and Administration. Baltimore: Paul H. Brookes.

Linder TW (1993) Trans-disciplinary Play-based Intervention: Guidelines for Developing a Meaningful Curriculum for Young Children. Baltimore: Paul H. Brookes.

McCollum JA (2000) Taking the past along: reflecting on our identity as a discipline. Topics in Early Childhood Special Education 20: 79–86.

McCollum JA, McBride SL (1997) Ratings of parent–infant interaction: raising questions of cultural validity. Topics in Early Childhood Special Education 17: 494–520.

McLean JE, Snyder-McLean LK (1978) A Transactional Approach to Early Language Training: Derivation of a Model System. Columbus, OH: Charles E. Merrill.

Mahoney G (1988) Maternal communication style with mentally retarded children. American Journal on Mental Retardation 92: 352-59.

Mahoney G, Boyce G, Fewell RR, Spiker D, Wheeden CA (1998) The relationship of parent–child interaction to the effectiveness of early intervention services for at-risk children and children with disabilities. Topics in Early Childhood Special Education 18: 5-17.

Miller JF, Leddy M, Leavitt LA (1999) Improving the Communication Skills of People with Down Syndrome. Baltimore: Paul H. Brookes.

NSW Ageing and Disability Department (1997) Recommended Practices in Family-centred Early Intervention. NSW Ageing and Disability Department.

Trevarthen C, Hubley P (1978) Secondary intersubjectivity: confidence, confiding, and acts of meaning in the first year of life. In Lock A (Ed) Action, Gesture, Symbol: The Emergence of Language. New York: Academic Press. pp 183-229.

Weitzner-Lin B (1997) A comparison of intentional communication in children who have Down syndrome with typical children matched for developmental and chronological age. Infant-Toddler Intervention 7: 123-32.

Yoder PJ, Warren SF, McCathren RB, Leew S (1998) Does adult responsivity to child behavior facilitate communication development? In Wetherby AM, Warren SF, Richie J (Eds) Transitions in Prelinguistic Communication. Baltimore: Paul H. Brookes. pp 39-58.

CHAPTER 5
Making inclusion work: improving educational outcomes for students with Down syndrome in the regular classroom

LORETTA R. GIORCELLI

Over the last half century, the education of students with Down syndrome in developed countries has been profoundly changed by so-called 'Integration initiatives' and more recently by the international inclusion movement. This has led to the gradual placement of students with special needs, i.e. children with disabilities, learning difficulties, behaviour problems and emotional disturbances, into the regular school either in regular classrooms or in special education classrooms within the regular school community (Lipsky and Gartner, 1989). The development of educational services for students with Down syndrome in most western countries, as for other students with special educational needs, could be summarized as one of progressive inclusion (Reynolds, 1990).

This inclusion movement, driven mostly by parents, social theorists and, to a lesser extent, by teachers, has seen a significant shift in traditional special educational services for students with Down syndrome. Twenty years ago most students with Down syndrome were educated in special (segregated) settings, whereas now, in most developed countries, the majority of these students are placed in the regular school. Students may or may not receive specialist support depending upon the funding basis of the school district. Despite these moves, some countries, states and districts have maintained special schools for students with special needs (residential or day schools) as part of a choice continuum for parents or for students whose complex needs are currently judged as best met in a separate, viable educational environment.

This significant educational change has been based on the principles of a *free and appropriate education* being provided wherever possible in the *least restrictive environment* and, wherever practicable, in the neighbourhood school. Such change has also been fuelled in Australia by a number of other significant factors. First, there has been a growth in parent advocacy movements made even more rapid by technology-driven ease of communication. This has seen the development of parental knowledge about their children's special needs. Informed decision-making by parents has resulted in a move away from traditional special/segregated residential and day schools to the regular classroom setting. Another consequence of this increase in knowledge has been a changed perception of the role of professional from that of decision-maker to adviser.

Shadowing the developments in the parent advocacy field has been the growth of self-advocacy/self-determination movements among people with special needs. These have both had a militant base (Morris, 1994) and been the expression of natural desire on the part of individuals with special needs to exercise autonomy in order to control, or share management, of their own affairs.

The education field has responded in many ways to these and other forces of change and re-alignment in the education of students with Down syndrome. First, there has been recognition of the learning differences as well as the learning potential of people with Down syndrome (Snell, 1988). Second, there have been ongoing attempts to more successfully implement inclusive educational practice for students with special educational needs as a result of disability discrimination legislation in many countries. Third, there has been a significant reconceptualization of Down syndrome as a result of the impact of more modern images of people with Down syndrome in the media and as characters in film, theatre and TV productions, leading to increased expectations and therefore a stronger focus on academic skill.

The concomitant educational context for these changes has been the development of the 'standards' movement, i.e. wholesale attempts to benchmark learning development in students at different stages and to quantify student successes as reflections of accomplishment along these predetermined scales. Along with this has developed, almost as a natural extension, a populist notion that schools can be ranked into 'league tables' with educational excellence measured primarily by exam/test results. This perspective does not take into account any measure of equity strategies or progressive educational changes taken by schools to accommodate the differing patterns of diversity represented in new student populations.

Another significant aspect of this context has been the move to generic support services in schools and the accompanying reduction in traditional withdrawal or separate 'special education' support services. For some students this has been a positive move. While Kauffman and Hallahan (1994) point to the lack of coherence in approaches to support provision taken by school districts to the disadvantage of many students with special needs, for some students with Down syndrome in effective inclusive environments, this has meant a move away from medical models. A consequence of this move is a change from pre-determined support to authentic student-centred, collabo-

ratively planned educational models of non-labelling support. The inclusion
of a range of students with special learning needs into the regular classroom
has also meant the recognition of dual disabilities in some students, with
regular teachers becoming aware of the blend of needs in some students, e.g.
those who are both deaf and learning disabled.

One of the impacts of the inclusion movement on the education of
students with Down syndrome in Australia has been the subsequent reduction in the continuum of services available to these students with the closure
of specialist schools for students with intellectual disability. The resulting
placement of students with Down syndrome into regular neighbourhood
schools has been characterized by school responses which have ranged from
'pathological' to 'generative'. In essence, schools can usually be placed at a
point on a change continuum which moves between these two responses.
The five points of the continuum can be described succinctly as:

- pathological;
- reactive;
- calculative;
- proactive;
- generative.

In the 'pathological' mode schools do not want to include the student with
Down syndrome and work actively or passively to reject the child and his/her
parents and fail to collaborate with other professionals working with the
child or the family. The challenges presented by the student are seen as
his/her 'pathology' or problem and the school personnel seek to justify why
they should not have the child placed or present in their school. Such schools
are often eager to redirect parents to other schools under the pretext of the
new school being better for their child.

In the 'reactive' mode schools, personnel feel they have been forced to
accept the student with special needs either by the disability discrimination
legislation of the country or state or by parental pressure. Here school
personnel will react or work with the child and family only when they realize
they have no choice and that placement is permanent.

In the 'calculative' mode, schools accept children who have diverse needs
and then set about finding out or calculating what needs to be changed or
done to accommodate that child in their community. Some mistakes may be
made where there is little experience among school personnel of the
challenges and the benefits of inclusive school practices but attitude, actions
and language are positive and non-discriminatory. Such schools may use a
disability awareness raising campaign or activities to help peers adapt to the
presence of a child with manifest disabilities.

In the 'proactive' mode, school personnel use the experience of accommodating diversity to their advantage and proactively plan for the physical, communication and instructional modifications that may have to be made for the child with special needs. They do not retest the child on arrival and have a policy of active social and academic inclusion of all students. They also reflect on the progress of their students and regard inclusion as a whole-school issue.

In the 'generative' mode, school personnel have arrived at the stage where they can successfully accommodate most children with special needs and are actively engaged in sharing ideas and suggestions with other teachers and administrators. They are collaborative and account to parents for their students' outcomes. They share responsibility and credit and are happy to be part of research projects related to the inclusion of students.

The question of what type of support is best for students with Down syndrome in the regular school setting continues to be a vexed one even in 'generative' schools. It is particularly so in 'pathological' schools where children with special needs are often physically placed in a class but receive the bulk of their curriculum from the teaching assistant(s).

One aspect of this problem has been the potential negative impact of adult proximity for students with Down syndrome supported as they often are in the regular school setting by specialist teachers, speech pathologists/rehabilitationists or by paraprofessionals in sometimes hothouse educational situations. Research suggests that the presence of additional adults in the classroom impacts on the students in terms of loss of space, loss of personal control, interference with peer interactions, loss of risk-taking ability, and a reduction in internal locus of control. For males there is also a risk of loss of gender identity because of the over-representation of female paraprofessionals in most regular schools (Giangreco, 1999).

In addition to the questions raised regarding the best use of extra teaching support, misperceptions about children, their families and the school community have the potential to impact negatively on the learning of children in regular classrooms (Brophy, 1986). For example, regular education personnel may overlook issues such as possible hearing loss, the learning status of parents, early intervention experienced and attentional difficulties in learning situations (Brookes and McCauley, 1984).

For these, and a host of other reasons specific to students with special learning and socialization needs, some researchers have maintained cautious opposition to what is called the regular education initiative, i.e. the concept that all students belong in the regular school, and that collaboration between special and regular educators will provide appropriate instruction for all students in the regular classroom setting (Kauffman and Hallahan, 1994). Kauffman and other long-time observers of the educational scene recommend that educators and parents should celebrate and utilize a variety of environments for the education of students whose needs differ markedly from those of their peers rather than assuming that the education available to students in the regular classroom is best for every student with special needs.

Educators and parents of students with Down syndrome are faced with difficult decision-making when it comes to the education of these children. Some districts and areas suffer from a paucity of adequate early intervention support and transition support to primary schooling for students with special needs, while others are characterized by a lack of literacy strategies specific to students with special needs in both primary and high school sectors. Students with special needs themselves are faced with a lack of role models with special needs in literacy, drama or social science, references needed for sound psychological development. The lack of involvement of adults with special needs and parents in educational processes is mirrored in the difficulty most regular schools have in setting up a disability-awareness raising program or in effectively supporting parents of children with Down syndrome in the school community.

The inclusion of students with Down syndrome into the regular school does however have some positive outcomes. These are, inter alia, the availability of a wider group of social contacts, an increase in diversity-awareness among peers, the potential for service learning (interdependency) for all students, the raising of articulated educational standards, an increase in opportunities for risk-taking, increasing self-determination and the use of brokerage models (to determine appropriate support for students in consultation with students themselves) and a healthy emphasis on students with Down syndrome as capable learners.

Kauffman and Hallahan (1994) acknowledge such positive outcomes of inclusion and embrace the move to more inclusive schooling environments (especially for those students with limited need for support too readily referred to special education by general educators in the past). They challenge educators, however, by suggesting that caution be displayed in moving to a uniform model for all students with special needs. They suggest this is especially necessary in those systems that provide alternative environments for gifted and talented students and gender-specific educational alternatives, i.e. educational systems that recognize difference in all students *except* those whose difference in learning needs is most obvious. They caution that unless total reform in the teacher preparation agenda occurs, teachers will continue to be overburdened with the diverse needs of large student groups. This, coupled with a lack of adequate specialist support, will create classrooms where all are at a disadvantage – that is, students with special needs such as those with Down syndrome, regular students, and their teachers.

In Australia, the slow creep in progressive inclusion means all teachers need to be prepared to help accommodate students with disabilities and learning/linguistic differences within regular school environments. In addition, special education teachers need to be prepared for consultation and teaming functions as well as for direct specialist teaching functions (Reynolds, 1990), and teacher education programs need to recognize the need for this broader training. (A distinction is made here between regular educators and special educators in that special educators are those regular educators who have both teaching experience and at least one year's additional study in the area of special education with a supervised practicum and therefore possess dual qualifications in regular – primary or secondary – and special education.) The knowledge base that constitutes the domain or discipline of special education refers to a range of technologies (access, communication and instructional), principles, skills and beliefs that support the teaching of children with disabilities, learning difficulties, behaviour problems and emotional disturbance as well as students with Down syndrome (Reynolds, 1990).

Recent research has highlighted this massive educational change and identified that there exists an overwhelming need for practising teachers to come to terms with the realities of mixed ability groups in order to make inclusion work. As Garnett (1996) describes, classrooms in schools today can be particularly challenging in numbers of ways for students who are especially vulnerable to particular facets of classroom ecology, i.e. children from impoverished backgrounds, children who speak English as a second language, children newly arrived from countries overseas, students in every classroom who have recognizable learning difficulties or attentional deficits, and children who have a definable disability like Down syndrome.

Garnett (1996) points out that today:

- Classrooms are crowded environments, arranged to maximize general, not close, observation of students.
- Classrooms are busy places, filled with varied interactions.
- Classrooms rarely operate in the flow of time but are mostly driven by clock time; yet despite time pressure much of student classroom time is spent either waiting or being interrupted.
- For students, classrooms are public arenas. The public spotlight can, at any moment, bare a child's failings or successes, making clear the official pecking order.
- For teachers, classrooms are private domains, rarely encroached upon for any length of time or depth of observation by another adult.
- Teacher talk predominates in classrooms, especially during times of intentional teaching. Student talk is minimal, especially during times of intentional learning.

- The instructional focus is largely at the activity level, with teachers expressing satisfaction when things are going well and students are enjoying themselves.
- Checking on students' performance is frequent, but uneven; probing an individual student's understanding, providing instructive feedback or monitoring individual progress is rare. Overwhelmingly, classroom instruction relies on whole-group instruction, accompanied by large amounts of loosely overseen seat work.

While many schools in Australia have adopted government policy in the area of integration and have developed more inclusive and sensitive learning environments, a common belief amongst school personnel is that including students with special needs is still fundamentally a matter of ensuring that the student is accepted socially (Gow, 1989). As Garnet (1996) found, teachers in general education classrooms aim for their students with special needs to be well accepted, for them to feel comfortable and to 'not stick out'. This translates into teachers not wanting to treat students with special needs differently – a pedagogical predicament, as the best approaches for dealing with the often complex learning needs of students with Down Syndrome essentially require either treating them considerably differently, or at least extensively differentiating the curriculum for them.

The lack of awareness of the specific teaching and learning needs of students with Down syndrome can result in a continuation of inappropriate non-inclusive practice occurring in regular classrooms today where teachers have not been initially or are not being currently trained to deal with children who have diverse special needs (Giorcelli, 1996; Watson and Giorcelli, 1999).

As Garnett (1996) observes in her research:

Fact 1: Teachers in general education classrooms, even those viewed as 'the cream', make minimal accommodations for students with disabilities and learning difficulties and tend to sustain only those they feel benefit their class.

Fact 2: There is a prevailing belief amongst regular educators that treating students differently is somehow detrimental – either bad for the individual, not good for the group, or both – voiced with particular concern for fairness.

Fact 3: In actual practice, neither instruction nor discipline is even-handed in classrooms, differing along lines of gender, race, class and disability or difference.

Fact 4: Different students are treated substantially differently in all classrooms. Some difference in treatment is intended but much is unintended, even unnoticed.

Fact 5:   One form of unacknowledged differential treatment is that students with learning difficulties receive decreasing academic challenges over time in regular education classrooms.

Fact 6:   Fairness, in the sense of sameness of instruction or equity of instructional care, or even in the sense of students being challenged to their potential, is not operative in most classrooms.

Fact 7:   Special educators, working in a regular classroom, are often forced to adapt to the prevailing focus on activity, activity flow, and the group's overall management and responsiveness. They become supportive regular classroom teachers often generalizing their advice in stereotypical rather than student-specific terms.

Fact 8:   Evidence suggests that special educators in regular classrooms, unless working in a true co-teaching model, do not maintain a student-specific focus, which suggests that there are cultural forces pulling negatively on classroom participants in inclusive classrooms even where schools have an active integration policy (Garnett, 1996).

For the purpose of helping schools struggling with the concept and the reality of moving to more inclusive school practices, *a framework for inclusive education* has been created. This framework has at its core (a) *knowledge of human rights* as an impetus to compliance with state or national laws outlawing discrimination on the basis of learning, physical or behavioural differences. It relies on teachers understanding the social justice implications of the principle of normalization upon which much change for people with special needs is based (Wolfensberger, 1972). It then focuses on (b) the *culture* of the school, measured by the inclusivity of the language used, actions taken and attitude displayed by adults towards students with special needs. The framework is further supported by the findings of the effective schools research both in the United States and in Australia (Comer and Edmonds, 1989; McGaw, Piper, Banks and Evans, 1993) with the inclusion of (c) *flexibility of management practices*. Such counter-hegemonic managerial stances need to be adopted in inclusive schools in the handling of the differing needs for consultation, staff development and problem-solving that staff members have when proactively seeking to improve the education of students with Down syndrome. Lastly but perhaps most importantly the framework for inclusive schooling practices depends heavily on (d) the *differentiation* made in the delivery of the curriculum and the *reasonable accommodations* provided in non-labelling, sensitive ways to students with special needs, including students with Down syndrome.

Arising from the application of such a framework in the evaluation of schools are the specific markers of inclusivity in any school that truly strives to make inclusion work for students with Down syndrome. These are:

- self-determination/brokerage, i.e. consultation with students;
- recognition of and exploration of disability-related cultural issues through disability-awareness raising or anti-bias programs;
- social skills training for students with Down syndrome in view of the differing social codes in many environments and situations;
- non-disability referenced language when referring to students with Down Syndrome;
- differentiation of instruction specific to students with Down syndrome.

Such differentiated provision in the inclusive classroom would also provide for reasonable accommodations specific to students with Down syndrome such as:

- interpreting (oral or modified signing systems when hearing loss is significant);
- simple note-taking;
- personal computers;
- alternatives to writing tasks in assessment;
- fatigue management;
- considerations of seating and instructor movement;
- peer awareness-raising strategies;
- home–school communication;
- consultation with support personnel;
- consultation with other professionals;
- co-teaching/collaboration between regular and specialist personnel.

The education of students with Down syndrome has made giant strides in the last 50 years. Access, communication and instructional technologies have led parents and teachers to the cutting edge of a brave new world. They are challenged to view this new world with optimism and commitment while the groundwork for such massive social change at the school level is still not securely in place in all schools. The needs for educators to break down old prejudices, to consult with adults with special needs and with parents, and to strive collaboratively to improve educational outcomes for students with Down syndrome, especially in literacy, are still with us.

The personal and professional re-conceptualization for such change is often slow and painful as we move from long-established comfort zones to the challenging, often uncharted terrain of inclusive schooling. Paraphrasing Tom West (1997) in his thought-provoking book *In the Mind's Eye,* the essence of inclusive schooling practices remains the adult's willingness (a) to change traditional educational practice and (b) to make reasonable accommodations in the classroom and playground for students who may think, communicate or generally perceive the world differently from others.

Acknowledgements

Portions of this paper also appear in the proceedings of the 19th International Congress on Education of the Deaf and 7th Asia-Pacific Congress on Deafness held in Sydney, 9–13 July 2000).

References

Brookes PH, McCauley C (1984) Cognitive research in mental retardation. American Journal on Mental Deficiency 88: 479–86.

Brophy J (1986) Research linking teacher behaviour to student achievement: potential implications for instruction of Chapter One students. In Williams B, Richmond P, Mason P (Eds) Designs for Compensatory Education: Conference Proceedings and Papers. Washington, DC: Research and Evaluation Associates. pp 121–79.

Comer JP, Edmonds R (1989) Fundamentals of Effective School Improvement. University of Wisconsin, Madison, WI: National Center for Effective Schools Research and Development.

Garnett K (1996) Thinking About Inclusion: A Teacher's Guide. Reston: Council for Exceptional Children Publications.

Giangreco M (1999) The tip of the iceberg: determining whether paraprofessional support is needed for students with disabilities in the general education settings. JASH 2: 281–91.

Giorcelli L (1996) An impulse to soar: silencing, sanitisation and special education. Australasian Journal of Special Education 1: 16.

Gow L (1989) Review of Integration in Australia: Summary Report. Commonwealth of Australia.

Kauffman J, Hallahan D (1994) The Illusion of Inclusion. Texas: Pro Ed Publishers.

Lipsky D, Gartner A (1989) Beyond Separate Education. Baltimore: Brooks Publishing.

McGaw B, Piper K, Banks D, Evans B (1993) Making Australian Schools More Effective. Canberra: ACER.

Morris J (1990) Pride Against Prejudice. London: Women's Press.

Reynolds M (1989) Knowledge Base for the Beginning Teacher. Oxford: Pergamon Press.

Reynolds M (1990) Educating teachers for special education students. In Houston W (Ed) Handbook of Research on Teacher Education. Association of Teacher Educators: Macmillan Publishing Company.

Reynolds M, Wang M, Walberg H (1987) The necessary restructuring and regular education. Exceptional Children 53: 391–8.

Snell M (1988) Curriculum and methodology for individuals with severe disabilities. Education and Training in Mental Retardation 23: 302–14.

Watson A, Giorcelli L (1999) Accepting the Literacy Challenge. Sydney: Scholastic.

West TG (1991) In the Mind's Eye. Buffalo, NY: Prometheus Books.

Wolfensberger W (1972) The Principles of Normalization in Human Services. Toronto: National Institute on Mental Retardation.

SECTION 4
LEARNING AND EDUCATION

Introduction

A theme common to most of the chapters in this section is the low expectations many people hold for the learning capacities of individuals with Down syndrome, and the subsequent effect this has on the learning opportunities offered to them. Jennifer Wishart's earlier chapter raises some of these same issues.

Sue Buckley and Gillian Bird have provided an overview of the work conducted at the Centre over the last 20 years. The research has had a strong focus on understanding the learning difficulties children with Down syndrome face, and on developing interventions to assist their learning. Speech, language and memory difficulties were identified by the group as the foci of their groups' research, and the majority of the work presented in this chapter deals with these issues. The usefulness of reading as a strategy to assist the development of language has been a core area of research for this group, and their results, including very recent work with preschoolers and adolescents, are presented. The importance of grammar and the role of vocabulary size in the development of grammar is discussed by the authors, using their own recent work as a basis.

In addition to their work on the cognitive difficulties of individuals with Down syndrome, the workers at the Sarah Duffen Centre have also advocated that inclusive educational experiences be available to all students. They present an overview of their work in this area and their data suggest that children benefit educationally from inclusive education, although they also identify some aspects of inclusion that require further development. The authors make a number of recommendations about where research might go in the future to extend the work that they have done or to resolve some of the remaining areas where results are inconclusive.

Literacy development in adults with Down syndrome has been a neglected topic, although there is anecdotal evidence that numbers of adults wish to continue their learning in this area after leaving school and are capable of doing so. For some adults, depending upon their schooling experience, literacy development may have been neglected during their formal education. For others, their failure to acquire literacy skills may reflect either a lack of interest, inadequate teaching, or delayed development. Whatever the initial reason for lack of progress in literacy activities, it is important that strategies that are effective for adult learners are developed and that services that provide a focus on literacy development are then provided. Christina van

Kraayenoord, Karen Moni, Anne Jobling and Kim Ziebarth report on a new initiative in developing the literacy skills of adults with Down syndrome. Their paper describes the principles guiding the teaching strategies used in the programme they have developed and the theories and evidence on which they are based. Although this is a relatively new initiative some evidence of effectiveness is already available.

The chapter by Sandra Bochner, Lynne Outhred, Moira Pieterse, and Laaya Bashash reports on a study of the numeracy attainment in adults with Down syndrome. The tasks used by these researchers reflect the real-life purposes of numeracy skills, and utilized time-telling and money-handling skills as the indicators of numeracy understanding. Comparisons were made across sex, age groups and school type. As the authors make clear, school type was a difficult variable to establish as most individuals in their sample had changed school type at least once. Results based around this variable therefore need to be interpreted very carefully; nevertheless the authors make a good argument that expectations and experience may account for the differences between those with better or poorer numeracy skills. Results relating to sex and money-tendering skills also need to be interpreted cautiously, since although there are consistent findings that males score better than females the differences between the two groups are, in all cases, small. As the authors point out, the difference is considerably larger if one outlying case is removed.

This paper will be encouraging to those engaged with teaching numeracy to children with Down syndrome. Clearly, many individuals will be capable of acquiring these skills. Bochner et al. have drawn out the benefit of real-life use of the skills, which has implications both for the salience of the skill and for its practice.

Chapter 6
Cognitive development and education: perspectives on Down syndrome from a twenty-year research programme

Sue Buckley and Gillian Bird

There have been several continuous themes running through the research conducted by the team at the Sarah Duffen Centre in the UK since 1980. One theme has been a desire to understand more about the cognitive development of children with Down syndrome and, specifically, the reasons for the typical cognitive delays. Central to cognitive development are speech, language and memory skills and this research group has published papers that explore the underlying difficulties in these skills in addition to developing and evaluating remedial strategies. A linked theme has been the exploration of literacy skills and the benefits of teaching children with Down syndrome to read for other aspects of their cognitive development. A third theme in our work has reflected our concern to optimize the social and educational learning opportunities of children with Down syndrome, particularly by inclusion in education. In this chapter, the authors will present the main findings of new studies in four areas – reading, speech and language, short-term memory, and developing inclusive education – and put them into the context of the cumulative findings of the Portsmouth research programme.

Reading

Reading research is probably the work that the team is best known for and this was a focus of the first research project in 1980. The possible significance of early reading instruction was highlighted in a letter to the first author from Leslie Duffen in 1979. Leslie had described the progress of his daughter Sarah on an early reading programme from three years of age. Sarah, at 11 years of age, had much better spoken language skills than the majority of children with Down syndrome and she was reading and writing for pleasure, as well as in school. Sarah was being educated in a mainstream secondary school, while almost all other children with Down syndrome at this time were in special schools for children with severe learning difficulties and reading was considered to be beyond their capabilities. Leslie was sure that early reading had been the key to Sarah's advanced language and cognitive progress.

The first Portsmouth study confirmed that many preschool children with Down syndrome could begin to learn to read from as early as 30 months of age and that this reading ability could be used to teach spoken language skills to the children (Buckley, 1985; Wood and Buckley, 1983). The team have continued to study reading at preschool and school level with longitudinal studies, providing information on rates of progress and levels of reading achievements as well as demonstrating the positive effects of reading instruction on language and short-term memory development (Buckley, Bird and Byrne, 1996; Byrne, Buckley, MacDonald and Bird, 1995; Laws et al., 1995).

Current work on reading includes two longitudinal studies, one with school age and one with preschool children. The first has followed 24 children with Down syndrome for five years in primary and secondary education and investigated their understanding of reading strategies as well as levels of reading achievement. The researchers also followed slow readers and average readers selected from the non-disabled students in the same classes or school year groups. The slow readers were matched with the children with Down syndrome on reading ability at the start of the study (Byrne et al., 1995) and the two groups made similar progress in reading during the first two years, indicating that the children with Down syndrome are reading within the range of reading ability of their peers in mainstream schools.

There are considerable individual differences in the rates of progress of the students with Down syndrome but most are steadily developing their skills and those with reading abilities at a 7- to 8-year level or above are able to use their phonic (letter–sound) knowledge independently for decoding new words and for spelling (Byrne, 1997; MacDonald, Buckley and Bird, 1997).

The second study recruited 18 preschool children with Down syndrome and 18 typically developing preschoolers, aged 3 to 4 years, into an early reading programme to be taught by their parents. The two groups made very similar progress in the first year. In both groups, some children learned many sight words (70 or more) and some learned only a small number. After 3 years, 11 of the children with Down syndrome and 16 of the non-disabled group could score on standard reading measures and there was no significant difference in the reading abilities of these two groups. The early readers with Down syndrome are now reading as well as their peers (Appleton, 2000; Appleton, Buckley and MacDonald, 2000). Clearly reading ability is a strength for many young children with Down syndrome and a very powerful tool for learning for them, as reading activities can teach new vocabulary and grammar, and improve discrimination and production of sounds.

The study of the 24 children in mainstream schools does not demonstrate a statistically significant link between independent reading ability measures on standardized tests and language skills as found in an earlier smaller study of 14 children (Byrne, 1997; Byrne, MacDonald and Buckley, in press). This is probably because in the earlier study, seven children were non-readers and most of these were in special school where the time spent on reading was probably less than for those in the mainstream schools (Laws et al., 1995). In the study of 24 children, all could score on a reading test and all were in reading instruction daily. This may mean that the key to the language gain is taking part in reading instruction rather than the level of independent reading achievement.

A recently completed study of teenagers with Down syndrome who have been mainstreamed all the way through school, provides evidence of a very significant gain in expressive language skills; a mean gain of 2 years and 6 months ahead of a comparable group of teenagers with Down syndrome in special schools (Buckley, Bird, Sacks and Archer, 2000). While some of this gain may be due to being immersed in a normal language environment, much of it may be due to daily supported reading and writing activities. The children record their work daily in written form, irrespective of independent reading ability, as they have a Learning Support Assistant to help them. This means daily exposure to reading and speaking correct grammatical sentences. Working on phonics and on spellings improves the children's sound discrimination and production skills, with consequent benefits for their speech intelligibility in everyday conversation. On the literacy measure (reading and writing skills) the mainstreamed teenagers with Down syndrome are 3 years and 4 months ahead of their comparison group in special school.

Case studies collected in Portsmouth suggest that the children who are introduced to reading between 2 and 3 years of age, as a consistent tool in a language teaching programme, make the greatest gains in language and in cognitive development and show excellent progress in school at 10 and 11 years of age, often reading at their chronological age level. This hypothesis should now be studied longitudinally, with a representative and sufficiently large sample. This study is possible now, as sufficient teachers and therapists working in early intervention would probably be willing to support parents to teach their children to read as part of their preschool intervention programme.

In the past, parents have often taught their children to read despite opposition from local professionals, providing important case study data but not a controlled research sample. The longitudinal study would require consistent teaching of reading in school as well as preschool years, and this has recently also become possible as a majority of children with Down syndrome are now fully included in mainstream primary education in the United Kingdom (Cunningham et al., 1998). In the inclusive classroom, the children join in the daily teaching of reading, which is now a priority in the UK National Curriculum and they join in the Literacy Hour each day. They are also supported to record all their curriculum work in writing. In special education, the quality and intensity of reading instruction does not match that available to the children in the mainstream classrooms, where they have Learning Support Assistants to ensure that the work is individualized to their needs.

The next important aspect of reading that needs to be researched is the development of reading comprehension. In our experience, most children have word reading and spelling abilities that are ahead of their reading comprehension abilities and teachers often report this to us as a concern. Comprehension difficulties could be linked to delayed language comprehension, but in the Portsmouth data sets, reading comprehension is almost always ahead of grammar comprehension (see Byrne, 1997). Limited auditory short-term memory spans in relation to chronological age may also cause comprehension problems. Studies are needed that explore the reasons for the children's reading comprehension difficulties and develop effective teaching strategies.

Speech and language

Reading is a language activity and our studies of reading have been inextricably linked to understanding the speech and language development of children and teenagers with Down syndrome. For most children with Down syndrome, speech and language develop very slowly and are more delayed than their non-verbal abilities would predict. Vocabulary is learned slowly and steadily throughout childhood but grammar presents a greater challenge and many teenagers and adults have only mastered simple grammar (Fowler, 1990, 1995, 1999; Gunn and Crombie, 1996; Miller, Leddy and Leavitt, 1999; Rondal, 1999). Most children with Down syndrome understand significantly more complex sentences than they can say (Buckley, 1993b; Chapman, 1997, 1999) and speech intelligibility is also a problem for them (Stoel-Gammon, 1997; Kumin, 1994, 1999). In our view, speech and language skills are central to the development of knowledge and of mental abilities (Buckley, 1993a, 1999a, 1999b). Words are the main means by which information is exchanged. The number of words an individual knows reflects their world knowledge. Typically, thinking, reasoning and remembering are all carried out using a form of silent language. It follows that significant delay in learning a language is bound to result in significant delay in the development of mental abilities, for any child.

For this reason, understanding the language learning difficulties of children with Down syndrome is a core focus of our research work and a series of small studies over the years, some separate from the reading studies and some linked with them, have provided data on the development of early language skills in children with Down syndrome. Observational data collected on video during the first early intervention project in 1980 to 1983 illustrated the children's ability to use gesture to communicate and to demonstrate understanding of events, and also drew attention to their specific speech and language impairment relative to non-verbal mental ability (Buckley, Emslie, Haslegrave and Le Prevost, 1986, 1993; Buckley and Bird, 1995a, b; Wood and Buckley, 1983).

Research at other centres in the 1980s reported a high incidence of hearing impairments in young children with Down syndrome (Cunningham and McArthur, 1981; Davies, 1985) and drew attention to their strengths in visual processing and visual memory relative to auditory processing and auditory memory (Pueschel, Gallagher, Zarter and Pezzullo, 1987). This work provided some possible explanations for the positive effects of making the language visual to the child via reading and signing as reported by the Portsmouth team. It also suggested that the significant language delay of children with Down syndrome might be due to the difficulties of trying to learn language from listening, rather than reflecting a general inability to understand and use language due to limited cognitive abilities.

Case study data suggested that the young children who were reading were mastering grammar that is usually not mastered by children with Down syndrome (Buckley and Bird, 1993). A training study working with teenagers also demonstrated that their expressive grammar could be improved with language interventions that included reading (Buckley, 1993b, 1995). A study in progress is investigating the effects of language teaching with and without reading activities for adults with Down syndrome (Jenkins, MacDonald and Buckley, 1999).

In the teenage study, the extent of the teenagers' phonological difficulties and auditory short-term memory difficulties influenced their rate of progress. In one of the memory training studies, improvement of short-term memory span was linked with significant gains in grammar comprehension (Broadley and MacDonald, 1993). Research investigating the significance of speech-motor delay and phonological difficulties for the delays seen in vocabulary and grammar acquisition still needs to be done. The Portsmouth team would predict that it is a major cause of the children's language learning difficulties.

A recently completed study has looked at the early vocabulary development of over 200 children and illustrates the typical relationship between vocabulary size and the development of early sentences and grammar for children with Down syndrome (Buckley, Pennanen and Archer, 2000). In typically developing children, once they have a vocabulary of over 250 words they begin to develop grammar. It has been recently suggested in the literature that this is not the case for children with Down syndrome, i.e. even when their vocabulary exceeded 250 words, they did not begin to develop grammar. However, these earlier studies have been based on very small samples (Bates and Goodman, 1997; Singer Harris et al., 1997). The finding of the link between vocabulary size and the development of grammar for children with Down syndrome has important implications for early language therapy, if a minimum vocabulary size of 250 words is necessary for sentences and grammar to begin to develop. At present some children with Down syndrome have not reached this point at 6 years or older. Very few parents will have been given a vocabulary list to work with to ensure that their child is learning the range of words that they need as fast as they could be, yet this may prove very helpful and a programme to teach an 800-word vocabulary is being developed by Buckley and colleagues.

A productive vocabulary of about 250 words may not automatically lead to grammar in all children with Down syndrome. Their short-term memory and phonological difficulties may hold some children back even when they have a vocabulary of more than 250 words. Here again, a longitudinal study is needed from infancy which provides parents with optimal support for vocabulary teaching and keeps records of hearing status, non-verbal mental ability and phonological development as well as of comprehension and production of words in sign and in speech.

The variation in the development of language skills in children with Down syndrome is very large. Some children are much more delayed than others. The range of spoken vocabulary for those of 5 years of age in our study of 218 children was from 8 to 649 words (mean: 294 words) and the range of vocabulary understood was 80 to 649 words (mean: 345 words). It is essential that this variation is investigated further as only when the reasons for it are understood, will it be possible to individualize therapy programmes to provide maximum help to parents and children.

A recent study still to be published has collected information on primary-age children, and has explored the links between language comprehension, language production and speech intelligibility in this group (Le Prevost, Buckley and Stores, 1999, 2000). Different profiles of strengths and weaknesses between these skills emerge for individual children and these do indicate different priorities for individual therapy programmes.

Short-term memory

Research at the University of York in 1987 (MacKenzie and Hulme, 1987) highlighted the specific delays in the development of short-term or working memory skills for children with Down syndrome. This memory system is used continuously during waking hours to hold incoming information for processing during all daily activities and interactions. Any difficulties in this system will influence all learning, including language learning, according to research with typically developing children (Gathercole and Baddeley, 1993; Baddeley, Gathercole and Papagno, 1998).

Studies conducted in Portsmouth have demonstrated the benefits of memory training in improving short-term memory function for children with Down syndrome, although lasting benefits of training seem to depend on continued support for learning and on being in a literacy programme (Broadley, MacDonald and Buckley, 1994, 1995; Laws, MacDonald, Buckley, and Broadley, 1995; Laws et al., 1995). A small study just completed in local primary schools has demonstrated the effectiveness of a computer program in improving short-term memory skills for children with Down syndrome, but the long-term benefits have yet to be evaluated (Buckley and Solomon, in preparation).

While some experts in the field are cautious about the possibility of improving short-term memory skills for children with Down syndrome by training, the Portsmouth team are not. The evidence that short-term memory skills in typically developing children are influenced by familiarity with material, by speech rate, and by reading progress, suggests that they develop in a dynamic and interactive way, influenced by and influencing progress in other cognitive skills (Gathercole and Baddeley, 1993; Gathercole, 1998). This supports the view that their development can be improved with direct training through memory games and similar activities. It also suggests that improvements in spoken language knowledge, speech fluency and reading instruction will influence short-term memory development. Further research in this area needs to consider and evaluate all these possibilities.

Developing inclusion in education

A survey of the development and social lives of 90 teenagers with Down syndrome conducted by the research group in 1986-87 (Buckley and Sacks, 1987) led the team to openly question the current practice of placing all children with Down syndrome in special schools. The academic achievements of this cohort were quite limited, few had the skills to move around the community independently and most were socially isolated out of school. These young people were going to find inclusion and participation in the community as adults very difficult. This study provided the most detailed set of information on the development of teenagers available at the time.

The findings of this survey added to the concerns that some of the team already had with regard to the potential negative effects on cognitive, linguistic and social development of isolating young children with disabilities from their typically developing peer group. The practitioners in the team were already encouraging inclusion in ordinary preschool provision for 3- to 5-year-olds. A further concern of the team was the effect of segregated schooling on the children's self-identity and self-esteem. Where a child has to take a special bus each day, with only disabled peers, while brothers, sisters and local friends go to another school together, this delivers a powerful negative message – that because the child has a disability, he or she does not belong with other children unless they are also disabled – and a daily reminder of being different and being excluded.

With the support of the Local Education Authority (LEA) and the expertise of a practitioner psychologist funded by the Down Syndrome Educational Trust, the team began to place children with Down syndrome into their local community mainstream schools in 1988. The LEA funded a Learning Support Assistant for each child and the schools and the team learned about successful inclusive practice as they supported each child.

The practical outcomes of this work, based on case studies, have been disseminated over the last ten years (Bird and Buckley, 1994, 1999; Buckley and Bird, 1998a, 1998b, 2000). A survey of the progress of 46 teenagers conducted in 1999 has provided a comparison of outcomes for teenagers of similar abilities but educated in mainstream or in special schools. The results provide powerful evidence for the benefits of being fully included in the mainstream school system and no evidence of any educational benefits of segregation in special schools despite the higher teacher–pupil ratio and the emphasis on practical skills in the special school curriculum (Buckley, Bird, Sacks and Archer, 2000).

The data are very informative as the two groups do not differ on measures of the skills or abilities which are most influenced by parents, such as independence in daily living skills, social skills and activities, and behaviour. This supports the assumption that the two groups of teenagers had similar learning potentials at the start of their school careers. Differences in school placement were due to education policy in the areas where they lived when they started school. The teenagers who attended their neighbourhood mainstream schools gained significantly in expressive language skills and in academic skills (reading, writing, arithmetic). On the expressive language measure they are $2^1/_2$ years ahead of peers in special schools, and in reading and writing they are 3 years and 4 months ahead.

The only measure that suggested a disadvantage for the included children is a measure of reciprocal friendship skills. The teenagers with Down syndrome are being supported in inclusive placements because they have had a lobby pressing for inclusion in the UK, while their peer group of children with a similar level of learning difficulties are still in segregated special schools. Therefore, although the other teenagers befriend them, perhaps they do not have the same opportunity to develop special friends and mutually supportive reciprocal friendships, except out of school. The implications of these findings are that all children with Down syndrome should be fully included in mainstream schools and so should their learning disabled peer group in special schools. There is no evidence to support segregated education in our data and the same conclusion was reached in 1998 by Cliff Cunningham and colleagues, though he does point out that no measures of self-esteem, friendships or happiness were available at that time (Cunningham et al., 1998).

The Portsmouth team do have some evidence on these issues. A study of popularity in inclusive junior school classrooms indicated that the children with Down syndrome were averagely popular overall, though less likely than average to be asked home to tea (Laws, Taylor, Bennie and Buckley, 1996). Interestingly, their popularity was not affected by poor language skills or by bad behaviour in the classroom. The first might be seen as evidence of appropriate allowances being made by the other non-disabled children in the class and helpful for the child with Down syndrome. However, the peers' tolerance of bad behaviour is not necessarily a positive or helpful response, as less tolerance from peers might help to encourage socially appropriate behaviour. Non-disabled peers who behaved badly in class were significantly less popular than those who behaved appropriately.

Another small study addressed self-concept and self-esteem in teenagers, half of whom were in special schools and half in mainstream schools. There was no difference in the self-esteem of the two groups, though this should be treated with some caution as available measures of self-esteem are far from ideal for teenagers with learning disabilities (Gould, 1998).

The next issues to be addressed in inclusive education are the development of social skills and friendships, and the development of number skills. In the UK, the experience of the Portsmouth team, from its involvement in research, support and training, suggests that teachers are usually confident in planning the curriculum and supporting classroom learning for children with Down syndrome. However, many children make much slower progress with number and maths than they do with reading and further research is needed here, especially as studies in Italy report that teenagers with Down syndrome can learn algebra (Monari Martinez, 1998), while in the UK this would be most unlikely to even be taught. Learning number is influenced by early experiences at home and by number vocabulary.

A longitudinal study of number development in young children with Down syndrome from 4 years of age is just being completed in Portsmouth and it has looked at parents' ability to engage their children in number teaching activities and the progress of the children in mastering counting and early number concepts. (Nye, Fluck and Buckley, 1999, 2000). There is a need for more research on the development of number and maths skills and of effective teaching methods for children with Down syndrome in primary and secondary education.

Evaluation of strategies to promote the development of age appropriate behaviour, thus reducing the occurrence of difficult behaviour in school, is needed. Similarly, evaluation of strategies to promote friendships and real social inclusion in school, which lead to social inclusion in an age appropriate peer group for leisure activities out of school, is also needed.

While behaviour difficulties in school and at home may arise for many reasons, one series of research studies carried out in Portsmouth indicates that daytime behaviour difficulties are linked to sleep disturbance (Stores, 1996; Stores, Stores, Buckley and Fellows, 1998a, 1998b). This link warrants further investigation and highlights the need to always consider physical health and well-being before looking for social and psychological explanations of children's difficulties.

The sleep studies indicated that the majority of children with Down syndrome are very restless sleepers, even those that do not wake during the night. In some children, sleep is disturbed by breathing difficulties, while others wake without an obvious explanation. Some sleep difficulties are behavioural and could be avoided by establishing good routines for bedtime, always putting children to bed at a fixed time and ensuring that children stay in their own beds throughout the night from infancy. However, other sleep difficulties may have physical origins which need investigating.

Many more teenagers are being included at secondary school level in the UK now, at least in some authorities, and are being supported by very positive staff teams. This will make longitudinal studies of the social and behavioural issues possible across the entire school age range.

Current conclusions

In our view, the key achievements of the first 20 years' research have been to demonstrate that we can have a positive effect on the mental abilities and developmental progress of children with Down syndrome. Specifically our work in Portsmouth has demonstrated:

- Most children with Down syndrome can learn to read to a level that is functionally useful; reading can have a significant positive effect on speech, language and memory, and therefore on mental development (even for those children who do not become independent readers).
- Speech and language are held back by specific difficulties linked to hearing, auditory processing, working memory and speech production

difficulties; making language visual by the use of signing and reading can improve both language and speech progress significantly.

- Working memory skills will improve with training but long-term benefits depend on consolidating the gains, being in an inclusive classroom in a normal language environment and being in a reading programme.
- Mental development is a process. Mental abilities, talking, thinking, reasoning, remembering, are learned, and they support one another in an interactive and dynamic way for all children. Central to all of them is the ability to develop language. If we work at supporting language, literacy and memory development for children with Down syndrome we then improve their mental development.
- Inclusion in mainstream schools and in all mainstream childhood activities in the family and community is essential for optimal progress, especially in speech, language and literacy development but also for social development and confidence.
- Sleep and sleep disturbance may be having a detrimental effect on the development of a significant proportion of children with Down syndrome, affecting both learning and behaviour, as well as disrupting family life, and should be receiving more research attention.

Acknowledgements

None of this work could have been done without the support and participation of children with Down syndrome and their families. The research team wish to record their thanks to them and to all the practitioners and schools that have worked with us on various projects over the years.

Staff and postgraduate students in the Portsmouth team have all made significant contributions to the work reviewed in this chapter, and are named below, past and present, in order of joining the team; other contributors mentioned as co-authors were undergraduate students in psychology.

Elizabeth Wood, Ben Sacks, Gilly Haslegrave, Linda Dalton, John MacDonald, Rebecca Stores, Brian Fellows, Irene Broadley, Angela Byrne, Patricia Le Prevost, Joanna Nye, Mike Fluck, Michele Appleton, Christine Jenkins, Christine Hamilton, Sally Gould, Glynis Laws, Brickshand Ramruttan, Mary Ramruttan, Freda Saunders, Tamsin Archer.

References

Appleton M (2000) Reading and its relationship to language development: a comparison of pre-school children with Down syndrome, hearing impairment or typical development. MPhil thesis, University of Portsmouth.

Appleton M, Buckley SJ, MacDonald J (2000) A three year longitudinal study of reading development among pre-school children with Down syndrome and pre-school typically developing children. Paper presented at 2nd International Biennial Scientific Conference on Down Syndrome, Toronto, October.

Baddeley A, Gathercole S, Papagno C (1998) The phonological loop as a language learning device. Psychological Review 105: 158-73.

Bates E, Goodman J (1997) On the inseparability of grammar and the lexicon: evidence from acquisition, aphasia and real-time processing. Language and Cognitive Processes 12(5/6): 507-84.

Bird G, Buckley SJ (1994) Meeting the Educational Needs of Children with Down's Syndrome: A Resource for Teachers. Portsmouth: University of Portsmouth.

Bird G, Buckley SJ (1999) Meeting the educational needs of pupils with Down syndrome in mainstream secondary school. Down Syndrome News and Update: 1: 159-74.

Broadley I, MacDonald J (1993) Teaching short-term memory skills to children with Down's syndrome. Down's Syndrome: Research and Practice 1: 56-62.

Broadley I, MacDonald J, Buckley SJ (1994) Are children with Down's syndrome able to maintain skills learned from a short-term memory training programme? Down's Syndrome: Research and Practice 2: 116-22.

Broadley I, MacDonald J, Buckley SJ (1995) Working memory in children with Down syndrome. Down Syndrome: Research and Practice 3: 3-8.

Buckley SJ (1985) Attaining basic educational skills: reading, writing and number. In Lane D, Stratford B (Eds) Current Approaches to Down's Syndrome. Eastbourne: Holt, Rinehart and Winston. pp 315-43.

Buckley SJ (1993a) Language development in children with Down's syndrome; reasons for optimism. Down's Syndrome: Research and Practice 1: 3-9.

Buckley SJ (1993b) Developing the speech and language skills of teenagers with Down's syndrome. Down's Syndrome: Research and Practice 1: 63-71.

Buckley SJ (1995) Increasing the conversational utterance length of teenagers with Down's syndrome. Down Syndrome: Research and Practice 3: 110-16.

Buckley SJ (1999a) Promoting the development of children with Down syndrome: the practical implications of recent psychological research. In Rondal JA, Perera J, Nadel L (Eds) Down Syndrome: A Review of Current Knowledge. London: Whurr. pp 111-23.

Buckley SJ (1999b) Improving the speech and language of children and teenagers with Down syndrome. Down Syndrome News and Update 1: 111-28.

Buckley SJ, Bird G (1993) Teaching children with Down's syndrome to read. Down's Syndrome: Research and Practice 1: 34-41.

Buckley SJ, Bird G (1995a) Understanding Down's syndrome: 1. Learning to talk. Videotape. Portsmouth: University of Portsmouth.

Buckley SJ, Bird G (1995b) Understanding Down's syndrome: 2. Learning to read. Videotape. Portsmouth: University of Portsmouth.

Buckley SJ, Bird G (1998a) Including children with Down syndrome: whole school issues. Down Syndrome News and Update 1: 5-13.

Buckley SJ, Bird G (1998b) Including children with Down syndrome: from the community to the individual. Down Syndrome News and Update 1: 60-6.

Buckley SJ, Bird G (2000) Down Syndrome Issues and Information for Teachers. Portsmouth: The Down Syndrome Educational Trust.

Buckley SJ, Bird G, Byrne A (1996) Reading acquisition by young children with Down syndrome. In Stratford B, Gunn P (Eds) New Approaches to Down Syndrome. London: Cassell. pp 268-79.

Buckley SJ, Bird G, Sacks BI, Archer T (2000) A comparison of mainstream and special school education for teenagers with Down syndrome: effects on social and academic development. Paper presented at 2nd International Biennial Scientific Conference on Down Syndrome, Toronto, October.

Buckley SJ, Emslie M, Haslegrave G, Le Prevost P (1986) The development of language and reading skills in children with Down's syndrome. Book and videotape. Portsmouth: Portsmouth Polytechnic.

Buckley SJ, Emslie M, Haslegrave G, Le Prevost P (1993) The development of language and reading skills in children with Down's syndrome, 2nd edn. Portsmouth: University of Portsmouth.

Buckley SJ, Pennanen T, Archer T (2000) Profiles of early language development for children with Down syndrome: the link between vocabulary size and grammar. Paper presented at 2nd International Biennial Scientific Conference on Down Syndrome, Toronto, October.

Buckley SJ, Sacks BI (1987) The Adolescent with Down's Syndrome - Life for the Teenager and for the Family. Portsmouth: Portsmouth Polytechnic.

Buckley SJ, Solomon N (in preparation) An evaluation of a Memory Training computer package for children with Down syndrome and peers with learning difficulties.

Byrne A (1997) Teaching reading to children with Down syndrome. PhD thesis, University of Portsmouth.

Byrne A, Buckley SJ, MacDonald J, Bird G (1995) Investigating the literacy, language and memory skills of children with Down's syndrome and their mainstream peers. Down's Syndrome: Research and Practice 3(2): 53-8.

Byrne A, MacDonald J, Buckley S (in press) Reading, language and memory skills: a comparative longitudinal study of children with Down syndrome and their mainstream peers. British Journal of Educational Psychology.

Byrne A, MacDonald J, Buckley SJ, Bird G (1997) Links between literacy, language and memory development in children with Down syndrome. Presented at 2nd International Conference on Language and Cognitive Development in Down syndrome: University of Portsmouth.

Chapman RS (1997) Language development in children and adolescents with Down syndrome. Mental Retardation and Development Disabilities Research Reviews 3: 307-12.

Chapman RS (1999) Language development in children and adolescents with Down syndrome. In Miller JF, Leddy M, Leavitt LA (Eds) Improving the Communication of People with Down Syndrome. Baltimore, MD: Paul H. Brookes Publishing Co. pp 41-60.

Cunningham CC, Glenn S, Lorenz S, Cuckle P, Shepperdson B (1998) Trends and outcomes in educational placements for children with Down syndrome. European Journal of Special Needs Education 13: 225-37.

Cunningham C, McArthur K (1981) Hearing loss and treatment in young Down's syndrome children. Child: Health, Care and Development 7: 357.

Davies B (1985) Hearing problems. In Lane D, Stratford B (Eds) Current Approaches to Down's Syndrome. Eastbourne: Holt, Rinehart, Winston.

Fowler AE (1990) Language abilities in children with Down syndrome: evidence for a specific syntactic delay. In Cicchetti D, Beeghly M (Eds) Children with Down Syndrome: A Developmental Perspective. New York: Cambridge University Press. pp 290-333.

Fowler AE (1995) Linguistic variability in persons with Down syndrome: research and implications. In Nadel L, Rosenthal D (Eds) Down Syndrome: Living and Learning in the Community. New York: Wiley-Liss. pp 121-31.

Fowler AE (1999) The challenge of linguistic mastery in Down syndrome. In Hassold TJ, Patterson D (Eds) Down Syndrome: A Promising Future, Together. New York: Wiley-Liss. pp 165-82.

Gathercole SE (1998) The development of memory. Journal of Child Psychology and Psychiatry 39: 3-27.

Gathercole S, Baddeley A (1993) Working Memory and Language. Hove, UK: Lawrence Erlbaum Associates.

Gould S (1998) Self concept in teenagers with Down syndrome. MSc thesis, University of Portsmouth.

Gunn P, Crombie M (1996) Language and speech. In Stratford B, Gunn P (Eds) New Approaches to Down Syndrome. London: Cassell. pp 249-67.

Jenkins C, MacDonald J, Buckley SJ (1999) Adults with Down syndrome: an investigation of the effect of reading on language skills. Fourth European Down Syndrome Conference, Malta, March.

Kumin L (1994) Intelligibility of speech in children with Down syndrome in natural settings: parents' perspective. Perceptual Motor Skills 78: 307-13.

Kumin L (1999) Comprehensive speech and language treatment for infants, toddlers and children with Down syndrome. In Hassold TJ, Patterson D (Eds) Down Syndrome: A Promising Future Together. New York: Wiley-Liss. pp 145-54.

Laws G, Buckley SJ, Bird G, MacDonald J, Broadley I (1995) The influence of reading instruction on language and memory development in children with Down's syndrome. Down's Syndrome: Research and Practice 3: 59-64.

Laws G, MacDonald J, Buckley SJ, Broadley I (1995) Long-term maintenance of memory. Down's Syndrome: Research and Practice 3: 103-9.

Laws G, Taylor M, Bennie S, Buckley SJ (1996) Classroom behaviour, language competence and acceptance of children with Down syndrome by their mainstream peers. Down Syndrome: Research and Practice 4: 100-9.

Le Prevost P, Buckley SJ, Stores R (1999) An evaluation of an early intervention programme for speech and language in children with Down syndrome. Fourth European Down Syndrome Conference, March, Malta.

Le Prevost P, Buckley SJ, Stores R (2000) Interventions to improve speech and language development. Presented at the 7th World Down Syndrome Congress, 23-26 March, Sydney, Australia.

MacKenzie S, Hulme C (1987) Memory span development in Down syndrome, severely subnormal and normal subjects. Cognitive Neuropsychology 4: 303-19.

Miller JF, Leddy M, Leavitt LA (1999) Improving the Communication of People with Down Syndrome. Baltimore, MD: Paul H. Brookes.

Monari Martinez E (1998) Teenagers with Down syndrome study algebra in high school. Down Syndrome: Research and Practice 5: 34-8.

Nye J, Fluck M, Buckley SJ (1999) Counting and cardinality in children with Down syndrome and typically developing children. Presented at the Fourth European Down Syndrome Conference, Malta, 10-13 March.

Nye J, Fluck M, Buckley SJ (2000) Children with Down syndrome counting with their parents. Presented at the 7th World Down Syndrome Congress, 23-26 March, Sydney, Australia.

Pueschel SM, Gallagher PL, Zarter AS, Pezzullo JC (1987) Cognitive and learning processes in children with Down syndrome. Research in Developmental Disabilities 8: 21-37.

Rondal JA (1999) Language in Down syndrome: current perspectives. In Rondal JA, Perera J, Nadel L (Eds) Down Syndrome: A Review of Current Knowledge. London: Whurr. pp 143-50.

Singer Harris NG, Bellugi U, Bates ED, Jones W, Rossen M (1997) Contrasting profiles of language in children with Williams and Down syndromes. Developmental Neuropsychology 13: 345-70.

Stoel-Gammon C (1997) Phonological development in Down syndrome. Mental Retardation and Developmental Disabilities Research Reviews 3: 300-6.

Stores R (1996) The pattern of sleep problems in children with Down syndrome and other learning disabilities. PhD thesis, University of Portsmouth

Stores R, Stores G, Buckley SJ, Fellows BF (1998a) Daytime behaviour problems and maternal stress in children with Down syndrome, their siblings, non learning-disabled peers and learning-disabled peers. Journal of Intellectual Disability Research 42: 228-37.

Stores R, Stores G, Buckley SJ, Fellows BF (1998b) A factor analysis of sleep problems and their psychological associations in children with Down syndrome. Journal of Applied Research in Intellectual Disabilities 11: 345-54.

Wood E, Buckley SJ (1983) Reading Skills in Pre-school Children with Down Syndrome video. Portsmouth: Portsmouth Polytechnic.

CHAPTER 7
Broadening approaches to literacy education for young adults with Down syndrome

CHRISTINA E. VAN KRAAYENOORD, KAREN B. MONI,
ANNE JOBLING AND KIM ZIEBARTH

People with intellectual disabilities have achieved levels of literacy that were once regarded by educators as unachievable. For example, in 1966, *The World of Nigel Hunt* (Hunt, 1982) became the first book to be written by a person with Down syndrome. There have also been a number of anecdotal accounts of individuals with intellectual disabilities becoming readers and writers (e.g. Anderson, 1995; O'Neal, 1991; Westby and Costlow, 1991).

Similarly, research evidence suggests that positive outcomes can be achieved for students with intellectual disabilities in the area of literacy (Katims, 1991; Katims and Pierce, 1995). There are an increasing number of studies that have indicated that students with Down syndrome can successfully be taught to read (Buckley, 1985; Buckley and Bird, 1993; Oelwein, 1995).

An examination of the literature shows that students with Down syndrome have been taught to read and write in a variety of ways. In this chapter we provide a brief historical account of the main approaches used to teach students with Down syndrome since the 1950s. This historical account suggests that there has been a broadening of the elements of literacy that have been the focus for teaching and a broadening of the ways in which literacy has been taught. We then report on an innovative teaching approach used in a research project designed to develop the literacy learning of young adults with Down syndrome. This approach is based on the social-cultural view of literacy learning which is increasingly gaining currency.

Approaches for teaching literacy

Educators have developed a range of approaches aimed at assisting students with intellectual disabilities to develop in literacy through learning to read,

write, speak, listen and view. Viewing refers to understanding graphic representations and still and moving images; it involves such processes as
analysing the technical features and visual content of film or video extracts.
Three of the major approaches used in the instruction of children with intellectual disability in the literacy domain are the behavioural, psycholin-
guistic/whole language, and more recently, social-cultural approaches.

Behavioural approaches

Behavioural approaches have been used to encourage the literacy development of children with intellectual disabilities, including those with Down
syndrome. Behavioural approaches involve structured procedures aimed at
ensuring that students learn specified responses or behaviours. When
applied to educational settings, the key elements of learning through these
approaches are frequent responding, progress in small steps, shaping and
positive reinforcement (Glover, Ronning and Bruning, 1990). Two common
behavioural approaches used with students with intellectual disabilities are
discussed.

Direct instruction

Direct instruction involves face-to-face instruction in which the teacher helps
the student to perform each step of a task, generally determined by a task
analysis. The teacher will tell, show, and model the skill and may use physical,
visual, verbal or gestural cues and prompts to assist students. Reinforcement,
such as encouragement and praise, or correction is then given.

The DISTAR Language Program (Engelmann and Osborn, 1976) is an
example of a well-known direct instruction reading programme. The
programme is based predominantly on imitating the teacher, with the teacher
shaping the desired response (Mercer and Mercer, 1985). In DISTAR, the
teacher first models a specific skill (e.g. saying a word), then elicits group or
individual responses at a fast pace, reinforcing appropriate responses or
correcting inappropriate responses.

The use of direct instruction to teach the skills of sight word reading and
decoding has been supported in a review by Adams (1990). Indeed, direct
instruction has been shown to be powerful in teaching sight words to
students in primary schools (Forness, Kavale, Blum and Lloyd, 1997) and
secondary schools (Schloss et al., 1995). However, following a meta-analysis
of research that examined studies of sight word instruction, Browder and Xin
(1998) raised concerns that it was not possible to demonstrate conclusively
that students participating in the studies understood the meaning or use of
the words they were learning, nor that they were able to apply their learning
to daily routines.

Precision teaching

Precision teaching (Lindsley, 1971) is another approach that has been used in the teaching of sounds and words. Precision teaching involves defining the behaviour to be taught (pinpointing) and observing and charting the behaviour (count and chart). The information from these two steps is then used to create aims and objectives. Next, a teaching procedure is implemented. Usually, this procedure is based on behavioural principles. Finally, progress is evaluated.

Typically, pinpointing involves an isolated target sound or word. The student is presented with a target sheet, and is required to say the isolated sound or word. For a writing task, the student is required to reproduce letters accurately. Tasks are timed with the focus solely on speed and accuracy.

A number of researchers have argued that precision teaching is effective in assisting students with learning problems and mild disabilities (e.g. Sparzo, in Sparzo, Bruning, Vargas and Gilman, 1998; Stump et al., 1992). Others point out that techniques such as precision teaching, which focus on sounds and words in isolation, do not pay attention to comprehension (Mercer and Mercer, 1985). Some research also suggests that combining direct instruction and precision teaching is effective in assisting students in various areas of learning, including reading (Maloney and Humphrey, 1982).

Psycholinguistic theories and whole language approaches

The view that the acquisition of literacy involved the teaching of a discrete set of skills and subskills that were to be mastered prevailed up to the 1960s (Edelsky, 1991; Luke, 1997). In 1965, Chomsky argued that pure imitation, upon which behavioural theories were based, did not explain the language development of children who were capable of producing new and interesting sentences. Furthermore, Chomsky pointed out that language comprehension could not be explained merely by stringing together the meaning of adjacent words. In order to understand complex sentence structures, children required special cognitive apparatus for inferring complex rules. The so-called psycholinguistic perspective arose from the work of Chomsky and other linguists. According to this view, children were innately predisposed to learn language, and were active learners who inferred rules of language and tested them out mainly on their own initiative. This was a dramatic departure from the behaviourist view (Pearson and Stephens, 1998).

The work of Goodman (1989) and others (e.g., Clay, 1972a; Holdaway, 1979; Smith, 1973) led to the emergence of whole language approaches to literacy instruction. According to this approach, students acquire the skills of written language in the same way as they do oral language. That is, just as children develop language skills through natural interactions with the linguistic environment, so too the skills of literacy will develop when a student is surrounded by an environment rich in print and opportunities to use print in authentic situations (Goodman, 1989). Whole language approaches focus on deriving meaning from words and texts, rather than on learning sounds and words as skills and subskills, characteristic of the behavioural approaches.

The concept of emergent literacy came about as educators (and parents) recognized the importance of the social context of learning and of learning through meaningful activities. Emergent literacy is 'the gradual and natural emergence of literacy competence, which occurs in tandem with spoken language learning from birth, through active participation in everyday language and literacy events' (Watkins and Bunce, 1996: 193). Key character- istics of programmes that seek to develop emergent literacy behaviours include the creation of a print-rich environment, everyday experiences with print, the development of reading and writing together, and supportive oral language interactions with adults (Sulzby, 1986; Teale and Sulzby, 1989).

A number of researchers have explored the literacy learning of students with intellectual disabilities from an emergent literacy perspective. Perhaps the most significant of these has been the research of Katims (1990, 1991, 1994). Katims found that the literacy development of children with intellec- tual disabilities can be enhanced through programs based on emergent literacy principles. More recently, in their study of a home-based emergent literacy programme, Saint-Laurent, Giasson and Couture (1998) found that there was a statistically significant change in the pretend reading of preschoolers with intellectual disabilities. While there were no other statisti- cally significant differences in performance among the children, the authors argue that their program had a 'modest but promising effect' (1998: 278).

Social-cultural approaches

The most recent contribution to understanding literacy comes from the social-cultural perspective. We are not aware of any research that has taken this perspective in assisting students with intellectual disabilities to develop literacy, except the research that we will report on below. Elements of the approach have, however, been undertaken in the work of Erickson and Koppenhaver (1995, 1998).

The social-cultural view recognizes that language is a social practice. This means that literacy is seen as a social construction with learners encouraged to think critically as they read, write, listen, speak and view (Freebody and Luke, 1990; Gee, 1996a; Luke and Freebody, 1999).

The theoretical underpinning of the social-cultural view comes from Vygotsky (1968). One of Vygotsky's major contributions to the under- standing of literacy as social is the concept that our higher mental functioning derives from our social communication. He argued that language is the foundation for all cognitive processes, including self-awareness, concept formation and problem solving. According to Vygotsky, learning takes place within an individual's zone of proximal development. The zone of proximal development refers to the area between the level where a student is currently achieving, and the level that can be achieved if there is assistance from someone else, such as a sympathetic adult. Children take the language used during these interactions, internalize it and use it to shape their own thinking.

The social-cultural perspective uses an holistic approach to literacy instruction and draws on a wide range of learning strategies in a literacy-rich environment. These approaches may involve shared discussions about text, brainstorming and scaffolding as well as guiding critical thinking, challenging of perspectives and engaging metacognition (Stewart-Dore, 1996). The approaches also often involve the integrated use of visual, as well as traditional print and media literacies (Luke and van Kraayenoord, 1998).

While behaviourist and psycholinguistic theories and whole language approaches continue to be used in the teaching of reading to people with intellectual disabilities, we would argue that the sole reliance on these approaches does not allow for practices that acknowledge and apply more recent theories of literacy, such as the social-cultural theories of literacy (Gee, 1996b; Luke, 1995; Luke and Freebody, 1997; Santa Barbara Discourse Group, 1994). Furthermore, we suggest that 'what counts' as literacy for people with intellectual disabilities, particularly young adults who live in 'New Times' has changed. Current views of literacy now acknowledge and embrace social and cultural practices. Literacy learning for young people with intellectual disabilities involves reading, writing, speaking, listening to, and viewing multiple texts (e.g. videos, computer games, popular culture, as well as functional texts such as safety signs and documents for daily living). Consequently, the teaching approaches and strategies used with this population need to be broadened in line both with current shifts in our understanding of what literacy is and with changes in society.

Social-cultural approaches may still incorporate elements of the behavioural and whole language approaches that have been effective in the past, but these elements are used within a wider construction of literacy as a social-cultural practice. In LATCH-ON, which is described below, we continue to draw on elements of these earlier models as well as using a range of strategies that focus on socially and personally relevant literacy development. To state our point explicitly: the social-cultural approaches do not preclude the use of a technique such as direct instruction but these approaches frame such a technique within a more all-encompassing view of literacy as well as placing the technique in a wider, more socially just and personally relevant set of practices.

The programme described below was designed to reflect social-cultural approaches to the teaching of literacy. It was considered that these approaches would enhance and challenge students to use their literacy skills across adult environments in numerous ways.

LATCH-ON (Literacy and Technology Hands-On)

LATCH-ON (Literacy and Technology Hands-On: Moni and Jobling, 2000) is a programme of literacy instruction specifically aimed at young people with Down syndrome who have recently left school. LATCH-ON was established at the University of Queensland in 1998. The programme arises out of findings related to cognitive development beyond childhood into adolescence and other developmental data obtained from the Down Syndrome Research Program (Crombie and Gunn, 1998). It is not an intervention programme but the continuation of literacy instruction into young adulthood using current effective approaches to literacy teaching. This approach is supported by research that suggests that individuals with Down syndrome may be more developmentally ready to learn when they reach young adulthood (Fowler, Doherty and Boynton, 1995). The programme attempts to build on the students' strengths and to remediate some of their weaknesses. Twenty-one students have participated in the programme. Six students graduated in December 1999, after two years of tuition. In 2000, the third year of operation, two groups of students (a total of 13 students) attended the programme for two full days each week.

Aims and features of the programme

In keeping with current theories, the definition of literacy that underpins the programme is one that has been commonly adopted in Australian educational systems:

> Literacy involves the integration of reading, writing, listening, speaking and critical thinking. It includes cultural knowledge which enables a speaker, writer or reader to use language appropriate to different social situations.
> (Department of Education, Employment and Training, 1991: 4)

This definition includes more than traditional reading and writing, as it focuses on the social and cultural nature of language use. It also includes a broader definition of the literacy skills of young adults than that offered by literacy programmes that focus on functional literacy skills. This broader repertoire of literacy practices that young adults need to develop during their engagement with texts includes those suggested by Freebody and Luke (1990) in their Four Resources Model of possible literacy practices.

These practices, elaborated further by Luke and Freebody (1999), include developing skills so that the young adults can recognize and decode the fundamental features of written text which include sounds, letters, spelling and language conventions. The second aspect of practice is being able to participate in the meaning of texts, that is, to understand and compose texts that have meaning both for the authors and in the wider community. Third, young adults need to be able to use and act on the texts they read, speak and compose. Finally, young adults need to be able to critique and analyse texts, particularly those related to popular culture, in their communities.

Consistent with this view of literacy as social-cultural practice, the main aims of the programme are to develop the young adults' abilities to communicate in written, oral and visual mediums in a range of social contexts. Literacy is constructed as a desirable and valued aspect in the students' continuing quality of life. This stance is in contrast to functional approaches to literacy evident in transition and other post-school literacy programmes (Riches, 1996). In the teaching and learning activities technology-based learning is linked with literacy teaching. For example, using e-mail assists students to use their literacy skills to foster friendships in the wider community. The university context of the programme is important both in enhancing the self-esteem of the young adults, who see themselves as studying, and in enabling them to interact with their peers in tutoring activities.

Teaching strategies

A range of teaching strategies have been created and implemented in the programme to develop this broad repertoire of literacy practices. Four teaching strategies that draw on elements of the social-cultural theories of literacy learning and that teachers have found to be effective are described in the next section of the chapter. These strategies focus specifically on scaffolding the acquisition of literacy in all language modes.

Photographs

Photographs are a useful resource for supporting students' literacy because they are visual representations of important, known events in family life. As such they provide meaningful individualized scaffolds for developing literacy. Photos are used to ask students to tell stories, and to sequence events; for example, of a holiday, at weddings or birthdays. Writing activities include writing captions/bubbles for photos, writing about photos, and naming the people and places in the pictures. Reading activities can include reading back the story or the captions and recognizing names. The students read and re-read about themselves based on photos, thus providing opportunities for repetitive practice and revision.

Joint construction of written texts

Students with emerging or limited literacy skills often find the idea of writing challenging. When the students in the programme try to write independently the writing is very short and sometimes unconnected. In class the teachers write with the students to share the cognitive burden and to extend their writing. This involves asking them questions about what they want to say, writing a sentence each, asking the students to dictate what they want to say and then reading it back with questions such as ' Is this right?', 'Is this what you want to say?' and 'Does this make sense?'. The teachers have found it is important to write down exactly the words that the students say, so that they retain ownership of the writing. In this way they are more able to read their own written words.

Shared reading

Shared reading follows the same principles as the joint construction of texts. In this instance however, the teachers work with the students towards a joint construction of meaning from understanding a text. Reading something together may involve reading a sentence, or reading a paragraph or a page in turn. This helps to maintain the flow and pleasure of the story without overloading the students' thinking or placing an unnecessary burden upon them, which may reduce their enjoyment of the task. Shared reading also involves asking questions about the title of a story, the pictures and what is happening. The teachers have observed that while the students are able to decode many of the texts they read, often they do not understand what they have just read. Asking questions to check that the students understand what they are reading is probably the most important strategy the teachers of the programme use to develop comprehension. Later, with this modelling, it is hoped that students will use this strategy independently.

Purposeful reading, writing and talking

For any reading or writing activity to be effective, it must be purposeful and have real outcomes for the students. Copying out lists of words or sentences may assist in improving letter formation and develop some sight vocabulary but unless the words are used in an activity that means something to the students, it is unlikely a real understanding of how to use these words will develop. Purposeful writing can be as simple as writing a shopping list, a birthday greeting, a name in a book, a birthday wish list, or an address to write to their favourite pop star.

A tape recorder is a valuable aid to developing oral language and can also be used to enhance reading and writing. An audiotape can be played back, a speech can be rehearsed, and the tape acts as a memory aid. Reading can be taped, played back and rehearsed to develop fluency. This works particularly well if the tape goes home or to a relative as part of a taped letter where instead of writing, the students can record their news. Recorded material can also be used to help with writing. The teachers have found that students lose track of their stories as they try to transpose them from oral language to written text. Using a tape of the story helps them to remember the sequence of events more clearly.

Preliminary results

Quantitative and qualitative data have been collected from students who have been in the programme for the last two years. As this project did not use a comparison group, the results are descriptive rather than experimental. Several instruments were used in the pre- and post-programme assessments of literacy. These include the Neale Reading Analysis–Revised (1988), Woodcock Reading Mastery Test–Revised (1987), Concepts of Print (Clay, 1972b), and PPVT-R (Dunn and Dunn, 1981). Samples of language development have been collected during oral activities using videotapes. Portfolios of the students' written work have also been compiled. In this chapter, trends from the data collected using the Neale Reading Analysis–Revised are reported.

The initial analysis shows some gains in students' reading based on the normative aspects of this test. Of the six students who graduated in 1999, all made gains in their reading rate. These gains ranged from four months to four years, with four students making gains of over three years. Increases in accuracy ranged from one month to 20 months with three students making gains of over 12 months. The average gain was 14.4 months. Finally, gains were also made in the students' comprehension. The smallest gain was one month, the highest gain was 15 months and the average gain was 8.8 months.

Conclusion

Our historical account of the development of approaches for teaching literacy to students with intellectual disabilities, including those with Down syndrome, has focused on three different approaches. While the first two approaches have been successful, in and of themselves, in assisting students with Down syndrome to learn to read and write, the social-cultural approach which is used in the LATCH-ON programme is a powerful addition to the field.

Strategies which move beyond those used in behavioural and psycholinguistic/whole language approaches to more social-cultural approaches encourage students with Down syndrome to read, write, listen, speak and view in personally and socially relevant ways.

The preliminary findings from the LATCH-ON programme support the view that when young adults with Down syndrome are provided with opportunities to broaden their literacy education through appropriate teaching and learning strategies, they continue to develop and improve their language and literacy skills. In addition to this increase in skill, parents and other observers of the young adults have noted the young adults have increased in self-confidence and are able to participate more fully in their social communities.

Acknowledgements

Elements of the first part of this chapter appeared in Part 2, Chapter 4, of 'Literacy and Students with Disabilities' written by K. Ziebarth and C.E. van Kraayenoord in a report to the Department of Education, Training and Youth Affairs entitled *Literacy, Numeracy and Students with Disabilities* by van Kraayenoord, Elkins, Palmer et al. (2000). This report is available from http://www.gu.edu.au/school/cls/cler.

References

Adams MJ (1990) Beginning to Read: Thinking and Learning About Print. Cambridge, MA: MIT Press.

Anderson N (1995) No, Belinda set everything up . . . Quick. Journal of the Queensland Society for Information Technology in Education 54: 8–12.

Browder DM, Xin YP (1998) A meta-analysis and review of sight word research and its implications for teaching functional reading to individuals with moderate and severe disabilities. Journal of Special Education 32: 130–53.

Buckley S (1985) Attaining basic educational skills: reading, writing and number. In Lane D, Stratford B (Eds) Current Approaches to Down's Syndrome. Eastbourne: Holt, Rinehart and Winston. pp 315–43.

Buckley S, Bird G (1993) Teaching children with Down's syndrome to read. Down's Syndrome: Research and Practice 1: 34–9.

Chomsky N (1965) Aspects of the Theory of Syntax. Cambridge, MA: MIT Press.

Clay M (1972a) Reading: The Patterning of Complex Behaviour. Auckland: Heinemann.

Clay M (1972b) The Early Detection of Reading Difficulties: A Diagnostic Survey with Recovery Procedures. Auckland: Heinemann.

Crombie M, Gunn P (1998) Early intervention, families, and adolescents with Down syndrome. International Journal of Disability, Development, and Education: 45: 253–81.

Department of Employment, Education, Training and Youth Affairs (1991) Australian Language and Literacy Policy. Canberra: Author.

Dunn LM, Dunn LM (1981) Peabody Picture Vocabulary Test – Revised. Circle Pines, MN: American Guidance Service.

Edelsky C (1991) With Literacy and Justice for All: Rethinking the Social in Language Education. Bristol, PA: Falmer Press.

Engelmann S, Osborn J (1976) DISTAR: An Instructional System. Chicago: Science Research Associates.

Erickson KA, Koppenhaver DA (1995) Developing a literacy program for children with severe disabilities. The Reading Teacher 48: 676–84.

Erickson KA, Koppenhaver DA (1998) Using the 'write talk-nology' with Patrik. Teaching Exceptional Children 31: 58-64.

Forness SR, Kavale KA, Blum IM, Lloyd JW (1997) Mega-analysis of meta-analyses: what works in special education and related services. Teaching Exceptional Children 29: 4-9.

Fowler AE, Doherty BJ, Boynton L (1995) Basis of reading skills in young adults with Down syndrome. In Nadel L, Rosenthal D (Eds) Down Syndrome: Living and Learning in the Community. New York: Wylie-Liss. pp 182-96.

Freebody P, Luke A (1990) Literacies' programs: debates and demands in cultural context. Prospect: A Journal of Australian TESOL 11: 7-16.

Gee JP (1996a) Literacy and social minds. In Bull G, Anstey M (Eds) The Literacy Lexicon. Sydney: Prentice Hall. pp 5-16.

Gee JP (1996b) Social Linguistics and Literacies. London: Taylor and Francis.

Glover JA, Ronning RR, Bruning RH (1990) Cognitive Psychology for Teachers. New York: Macmillan Publishing Co.

Goodman KA (1989) Whole-language research: foundations and development. Elementary School Journal 90: 207-21.

Holdaway D (1979) The Foundations of Literacy. Gosford, NSW: Ashton Scholastic.

Hunt N (1982) The World of Nigel Hunt: The Diary of a Mongoloid Youth. Norwich, UK: Asset Recycling (originally published 1966).

Katims DS (1990) Project I.E.P. (Intervention for Early Progress): An emergent literacy approach to early childhood special education. Paper presented at the 11th Annual International Conference of the Young Adult Institute of Developmental Disabilities, New York, April.

Katims DS (1991) Emergent literacy in early childhood special education: curriculum and instruction. Topics in Early Childhood Special Education 11: 69-84.

Katims DS (1994) Emergence of literacy in preschool children with disabilities. Learning Disability Quarterly 17: 58-69.

Katims DS, Pierce PL (1995) Literacy-rich environments and transition of young children with special needs. Topics in Early Childhood Special Education 15: 219-34.

Lindsley OR (1971) From Skinner to precision teaching: the child knows best. In Jordan JB, Robbins LS (Eds) Let's Try Doing Something Else Kind of Thing. Arlington, VA: Council for Exceptional Children. pp 1-11.

Luke A (1995) When basic skills and information processing just aren't enough: rethinking reading in new times. Teachers College Record 97(1): 95-115.

Luke A (1997) Critical approaches to literacy. In Edwards V, Corson D (Eds) The Encyclopedia of Language and Education, Vol 2: Literacy. Dordrecht, The Netherlands: Kluwer Academic Publishers. pp 143-51.

Luke A, Freebody P (1997) Social practices of reading. In Muspratt S, Luke A, Freebody P (Eds) Constructing Critical Literacies: Teaching and Learning Textual Practice. Cresskill, NJ: Hampton Press Inc. pp 185-225.

Luke A, Freebody P (1999) A map of possible practices: further notes on the Four Resources Model. Practically Primary 4(2): 5-8.

Luke A, van Kraayenoord CE (1998) Babies, bathwaters and benchmarks. Curriculum Perspectives 18(3): 55-61.

Maloney M, Humphrey JE (1982) The Quinte Centre: a successful venture in behavioral education. Behavioral Educator 4: 1-3.

Mercer CD, Mercer AR (1985) Teaching Students with Learning Problems (2nd ed). Columbus, OH: Charles E. Merrill Publishing Co.

Moni KB, Jobling A (2000) LATCH-ON: a program to develop literacy in young adults with Down syndrome. Journal of Adolescent and Adult Literacy 44: 40-9.

Neale MD (1988) Neale Analysis of Reading Ability - Revised. Hawthorn, VIC: Australian Council for Educational Research.

Oelwein PL (1995) Teaching Reading to Children with Down Syndrome: A Guide for Parents and Teachers. Bethesda, MD: Woodbine House, Inc.

O'Neal S (1991) Leadership in the language arts: Dear principal, please let my special education child read and write. Language Arts 68: 417-23.

Pearson PD, Stephens D (1998) Learning about literacy: a 30-year journey. In Weaver C (Ed) Reconsidering a Balanced Approach to Reading. Urbana, IL: National Council of Teachers of English.

Riches V (1996) A review of transition from school to community for students with disabilities in NSW Australia. Journal of Intellectual and Developmental Disability 21: 71-88.

Saint-Laurent L, Giasson J, Couture C (1998) Emergent literacy and intellectual disabilities. Journal of Early Intervention 21: 267-81.

Santa Barbara Discourse Group (1994) Constructing literacy in classrooms. In Ruddell RB, Ruddell MR, Singer H (Eds) Theoretical Models and Processes of Reading (4th ed). Newark, DE: International Reading Association. pp 124-54.

Schloss PJ, Alper S, Young H, Arnold-Reid D, Aylward M, Dudenhoeffer S (1995) Acquisition of functional sight words in community-based recreation settings. Journal of Special Education 29: 84-96.

Smith F (1973) Psycholinguistics and Reading. New York: Holt, Rinehart and Winston.

Sparzo FJ, Bruning R, Vargas JS, Gilman DA (1998) Educational problems for the 21st century, part II: Teaching. Contemporary Education (Online) 70(1). Available at: http://proquest.umi.com.

Stewart-Dore N (1996) Literacy strategies for learning. In Bull G, Anstey A (Eds) The Literacy Lexicon. Sydney: Prentice Hall. pp 127-44.

Stump CS, Lovitt TC, Fister S, Kemp K, Moore R, Schroeder B (1992) Vocabulary intervention for secondary-level youth. Learning Disability Quarterly 15: 207-22.

Sulzby E (1986) Writing and reading: signs of oral and written language organization in the young child. In Teale W, Sulzby E (Eds) Emergent Literacy: Writing and Reading. Norwood, NJ: Ablex Publishing Company. pp 50-89.

Teale W, Sulzby E (1989) Emergent literacy: new perspectives. In Strickland D, Morrow L (Eds) Emerging Literacy: Young Children Learn to Read and Write. Newark, DE: International Reading Association. pp 1-15.

Vygotsky LS (1968) Mind in Society: The Development of Higher Psychological Processes. Cambridge, MA: Harvard University Press.

Watkins RV, Bunce BH (1996) Natural literacy: theory and practice for preschool intervention programs. Topics in Early Childhood Special Education 16: 191-212.

Westby CE, Costlow L (1991) Implementing a whole language program in a special education class. Topics in Language Disorders 11: 69-84.

Woodcock RW (1987) Woodcock Reading Mastery Tests - Revised. Circle Pines, MA: American Guidance Service.

CHAPTER 8
Numeracy and money management skills in young adults with Down syndrome

SANDRA BOCHNER, LYNNE OUTHRED, MOIRA PIETERSE
AND LAAYA BASHASH

Over the years since normalization became an accepted principle guiding the provision of services for people with intellectual disabilities, young people with Down syndrome have begun to live more independently within their local communities. To do this successfully, they need functional skills in basic areas of learning that include numeracy, and, more specifically, the money skills needed to cope with daily living tasks such as shopping and travel. This report is about a study in which information on aspects of these skills was collected from a group of young people with Down syndrome who completed their schooling in New South Wales during the 1990s.

Background to the study

In 1974, an early intervention program for young children with Down syndrome was established in Sydney (Pieterse, 1988) with the aim of providing parents and children with an individualized program that would maintain the development of the child as close to normal as possible. The early intervention program, and others that were subsequently established following a similar model (Pieterse, Bochner and Bettison, 1988) focused on developing the children's personal, social, cognitive and language skills. Reading skills were introduced as part of a language program, and subsequently other pre-academic skills were introduced, including numeracy, beginning with number recognition and rote counting to ten. A follow-up study of a group of nine children (age range 7–9 years) who were fully integrated at school showed that, on cognitive and social measures, the children were functioning in the mild rather than moderate range of intellectual development. Their reading and social skills 'were within the range of

93

variability tolerated in a regular classroom' (Pieterse and Center, 1984: 11). However, the children's achievements in the area of mathematics were found to be in the lowest percentile of the class.

The limitations in numeracy documented by Pieterse and Center (1984) have also been reported elsewhere (e.g. Berry, Groenweg, Gibson and Brown, 1984; Carr, 1995; Cornwell, 1974; Rynders, 1996, 1999). Rynders (1996) claimed that students with Down syndrome could become proficient in using basic arithmetic facts, but noted that they frequently had difficulties with tasks requiring more complex skills. He subsequently reported low mathematics grade-equivalent scores in longitudinal data on the Peabody Individual Achievement Test (Dunn and Markwardt, 1970) for a group of young adults with Down syndrome who had participated in the Minnesota/Illinois studies (Abery, 1988, as cited in Rynders, 1999; Rynders and Horrobin, 1996; Smith et al., 1984). Carr (1995) reported similar results; more than half of the young people in her sample could only recognize and count single numbers, skills generally seen among children in their first six months at school.

Counting skills and concepts of number in children with intellectual disability

A major question which must be considered when discussing number skills in people with Down syndrome concerns the extent to which their poor achievement is a function of limitations in cognitive ability or of a lack of opportunity to learn. To what extent are early levels of mathematical achievement based on understanding of number, measurement and space, and how much involves mechanical skills such as memorization of number facts? There has been considerable research interest in the development of children's counting and number skills. However, the number of studies regarding the emergence of these skills in children with intellectual disabilities is limited and the evidence they provide is conflicting.

Cornwell (1974) studied the development of numerical concept formation and abstraction in 38 young people with Down syndrome. Results showed some improvement, with increasing mental age, in identification and designation of objects in numerical units (e.g. 'Give me three keys' and 'How many keys are there?'), but in all cases, these skills remained low. Cornwell concluded that children with Down syndrome were able to learn counting as a rote task that did not necessarily involve acquisition of arithmetical concepts.

Gelman and Cohen (1988) were interested in Cornwell's suggestion, supported by their own work (Gelman, 1982), that children with Down syndrome could learn by rote but experienced difficulties in learning rules and more conceptual problem-solving strategies. They compared the performance of ten 10–13-year-olds with Down syndrome with typically developing preschoolers of similar mental age on a novel counting problem. Results showed that the two groups of children performed the task in qualitatively different ways. The preschoolers were more successful; they tended to self-correct their errors and understood subtle hints. Eight of the ten students with Down syndrome were less successful; they seldom spontaneously repeated a trial, did not self-correct and were unable to benefit from hints, even when the hints included explicit instructions or demonstrations of ways to solve the problem. Interestingly, two of the children with Down syndrome who had been classified at a pretest as 'excellent counters', performed the task in a way that was similar to the preschoolers. Gelman and Cohen concluded that the problems encountered by many children with Down syndrome in acquiring a language system may have been symptomatic of their difficulties in mastering symbolic material such as number words and other numerals. Such children were further disadvantaged by the limitations they experienced as a result of exposure to a restricted school curriculum, conclusions which were supported by Caycho, Gunn and Siegal (1991).

The development of counting and number skills in children with intellectual disabilities was the focus of a series of studies reported by Baroody (e.g. Baroody, 1986, 1988, 1995; Baroody and Snyder, 1983). In one study, Baroody (1988) designed an intervention program to find out if children with intellectual disabilities could learn number comparisons as a general rule, rather than only by rote as specific facts. The results suggested that rule-based number-comparison training could produce retention and transfer of trained skills by children with moderate intellectual disabilities. In contrast to the studies described earlier, Bashash and Outhred (1996) and Bashash (1997) also demonstrated that students with moderate intellectual disabilities (almost half of whom had Down syndrome) had an array of counting and number-understanding skills which could not have been acquired simply by associative learning. They also found no basic differences between the types of strategies used by the children in number-skill development and those reported in the literature for children with normal intelligence and the same mental age (e.g. Fuson, 1988; Gelman and Gallistel, 1978; Steffe, von Glasersfeld, Richards and Cobb, 1983). It seemed that the main difference in number-skill acquisition between these two groups was a matter of time, with the children who had moderate intellectual disabilities passing through the same stages as other children, but at a much slower pace.

Experience with number and mathematical concepts has been raised as an essential element in the acquisition of numeracy skills. It is probable that children in integrated settings would have more opportunities for this kind of experience than those in segregated settings, in part as a result of higher expectations for achievement by teachers (Center, Ferguson and Ward, 1988).

The specific aim of the study reported here was to examine the number and money management skills of a group of young adults with Down syndrome through informal assessment of simple number and money-tendering tasks. It was hypothesized that children who had received their schooling in an integrated setting would do better than those whose schooling was in a segregated setting. In addition, it was hypothesized that children born after the introduction of improved services for children with disabilities would have more opportunity to become numerate than children born before the introduction of these changes, and thus younger children would have more success on the tasks. Experience in an integrated setting and age are confounded, of course, with younger children being more likely to have received at least some of their education within a regular setting.

It should be noted that the study was not a rigorous statistical investigation of the factors identified here. This would have been impossible because of the small numbers involved, particularly in the oldest age group, coupled with the diverse range of skills represented in the sample group.

Method

The study reported here involved a survey of young people with Down syndrome living in Sydney in 1994-1995. Participants and, in some cases, their parents or carers took part in a structured interview and completed a series of formal and informal assessments of literacy and numeracy skills. Information related to numeracy is reported here. Data on literacy is reported in Bochner, Outhred and Pieterse (in press).

Participants

Participants in the study comprised 30 young adults with Down syndrome (14 female, 16 male) ranging in age from 18 to 36 years (median age 21 years). They were located through the New South Wales Down Syndrome Association. The participants were interviewed at home, with a parent or carer present (copies of the questionnaire that formed the basis of the interview and forms for ethical consent were sent prior to the meeting).

For the purpose of data analysis, the sample was grouped in terms of age and type of school attended (see Table 8.1). Three age groups were formed: youngest (18-20 years), middle (21-24 years), and oldest (over 24 years; actual age range 28-36 years). Two school groups were formed: integrated (this included those in a regular class as well as those in a special class within a regular school); and segregated (i.e. in a separate, special school). In fact, the type of school attended by participants was highly varied. Half had spent their

Table 8.1 Type of school attended for gender by age

Age	n	School				Gender	
		Integrated		Segregated			
		Male	Female	Male	Female	Male	Female
18–20[a]	12	1	5	3	3	4	8
21–24	13	3	3	7	0	10	3
>24	5	0	0	2	3	2	3
Total	30	4	8	12	6	16	14

Note The values represent frequencies of participants in each category.
[a] Represents chronological age in years.

first years at school in a regular classroom, but by the time they reached upper primary level the percentage in a regular class, or a special class in a regular school, had reduced to 37 and more than half moved from one type of class to another at least once while in school. On the basis of data collected on the type of class attended during primary and secondary school, participants were categorized in terms of the type of setting (integrated or segregated) in which they had spent most time. On this basis, 60 per cent were classified as having been educated in a segregated setting and 40 per cent in integrated settings (five in a regular class and seven in a special class within a regular school).

Most of the group lived at home while they were at school. However, six (five females and one male) were in residential care for some or all of their years at school and two had been in residential care from birth. At the time of the interview, most lived with their families but four were in group homes, under constant supervision, and one lived in a hostel which functioned like a nursing home.

Materials

Since the focus of the study was on the functional skills needed for daily living by people with Down syndrome, a set of tasks was designed which included the following.

Recognition of analogue and digital time displays

A card with a diagram representing a digital or analogue display (e.g. 8.00, 9.30, 12.00) was shown and the participant was asked 'What's the time here?'

Recognition of the value of coins and notes

5, 10, 20 and 50 cents, $1, and $2 coins and $5, $10, $20 and $50 notes were presented and the participant was asked 'What's this?'

Tendering of cash needed to buy a familiar item

Advertisements for seven familiar objects such as a bottle of soft drink ($2.95), a candy bar ($0.50) and a pair of sun-glasses ($15.95) were used to assess understanding of the purchase process (price of item, tendering an appropriate amount of money, and expected change).

Simple addition sums, four involving two single-digit displays

Using the context of shopping to introduce the task ('If I had $2 and $3, how much would I have?'), five simple addition sums were presented in written form, using a vertical format.

In addition, questions were asked during the interview about money management skills (e.g. payment of fares, purchase of snacks, etc.). The Peabody Picture Vocabulary Test–Revised (PPVT–R: Dunn and Dunn, 1981) and the Waddington Diagnostic Reading Test (WDRT: Waddington, 1988) were administered to assess receptive vocabulary and reading (see Bochner et al., in press). No tests of intelligence were used.

Results

In the following discussion, results achieved in time and money management tasks, and in the supplementary number tasks are considered in terms of participants' age, gender and educational backgrounds. Note that no test results are available for a 21-year-old male who declined to take part in the assessment procedures and a 31-year-old female who could not complete any time, money or number tasks.

Time

There were no significant differences by age and school type in performance on the tasks that involved reading three analogue and three digital clock displays. All the participants who attempted the time tasks were able to read the three digital time displays correctly. More difficulty was encountered with the analogue display; 21 made no errors with this task but two could not identify any of the analogue time displays, two recognized only the first ('7:00') of three items and four made an error on the half-hour ('5:30') display. This finding is not unexpected, since digital time can be read directly, whereas analogue time has to be interpreted from a symbolic representation. Comments noted during testing suggested that at least some of the successful group did understand the meaning of the time displays they read.

Money recognition

All the participants who attempted the money recognition tasks were able to recognize the value of the ten coins and notes shown to them.

Money tendering

Compared with their success in recognizing coins and notes, participants were less successful in the tasks that involved tendering money, particularly as the tasks became more difficult. Apart from one 19-year-old female, participants were able to identify the cost of all, or almost all of the advertised items (see Table 8.2). Only 18 of the group could show the actual coins and notes required to purchase the item from the array of money used in the recognition task, however. The rest could not do this task or gave only one correct response. Overall, data set out in Table 8.2 suggest that males did better than females on the money-tendering tasks, the middle (21–24 years) age group was more successful than the other two age groups and the integrated group did better than those from segregated backgrounds.

Three participants did particularly well on the money-tendering tasks. CW, a 24-year-old woman, made no errors while two young men (AB, aged 22, and ML, aged 23), only made errors on the final 'How much change?' part of the task. (In the tendering task, they used a 'rounding up' strategy, i.e. round the required sum to the next dollar and have a realistic idea of the change.) All three had work experience, travelled independently and managed their own money. CW had worked for six months, on full pay, in the kitchen at a city bank but had left as a result of health problems. AB had held a full-time job in a large insurance office for a number of years. ML had held a steady job for four years as a kitchen hand and waiter in a restaurant, initially full-time but more recently part-time, for health reasons. These experiences

Table 8.2 Mean percentage correct responses on the seven money-tendering tasks by sex, age and school type groups

Group	n*	Tasks			
		How much?	Show me?	Any change?	How much?
Gender					
Male	15	93	65	50	2
Female	13	78	49	28	9
Age (years)					
18–20	12	87	49	31	2
21–24	12	99	84	67	11
>24	4	86	21	0	0
School type:					
Integrated	12	94	73	60	12
Segregated	16	88	50	30	2

* Does not include 21-year-old male and 31-year-old female who did not take part in assessments.

probably contributed to their success in the tendering tasks. All three were in the middle age group; CW and ML had integrated school backgrounds, and AB was from a special school.

Total scores for the 28 money-tendering tasks confirmed that the males tended to perform at a higher level than the females (males: M=14.8, SD=5.6, range 5-22; females: M=13.1, SD=6.5, range 4-28; excluding the outlying score of CW, females M=11.9, SD=5.3, range 4-20). The mean score of the middle age group (18.4, SD=4.1, range 12-28: excluding CW, 17.5, SD=3.0, range 12-22) was markedly higher than that attained by either the youngest or the oldest groups (M=11.8, SD=5.4, range 4-20 and M=7.5, SD=3.3, range 5-12 respectively). The mean score attained by those from an integrated background (M=16.8, SD=5.3, range 7-28; excluding CW, M=16.0, SD=4.4, range 7-21) was also higher than the segregated school group (M=11.5, SD=5.6, range 4-22). Much the same pattern emerged when mean scores by age and type of school were considered (see Table 8.3), with mean scores for the integrated groups consistently higher than the segregated groups, and the middle age groups higher than the youngest and oldest groups.

Among the five participants from the oldest age group, four could recognize the value of coins or notes and read the cost of items in an advertisement. None could answer the more difficult questions about the money needed to buy an item and any change that could be expected, apart from one 36-year-old woman who attempted to answer the items that involved showing the actual money needed to purchase an item. She lived in a residential care situation and, according to her mother, had skills needed to use money but lacked the opportunity and interest ('she hated going into shops'). Within this group, one man was not working and the three women were at sheltered workshops (full- or part-time). Two lived at home and three in group homes or hostels. A 27-year-old male, who lived at home and had a full-time job, could recognize money and read prices. He had difficulty identifying the appropriate notes or coins to tender and had no idea about change.

Table 8.3 Mean total money-tendering score for age by school type (total correct = 28)

School	n*	Chronological age in years								
		18–20			21–24			>24		
		M	SD	n	M	SD	n	M	SD	n
Integrated	12‡	13.7	4.9	6	18.3	2.4	6	–	–	0
Segregated	15	10.0	5.5	6	16.6	3.6	5	6.0	4.4	4

* Does not include outlier scores (CW).
‡ Does not include 21-year-old male and 31-year-old female who did not take part in assessments.

However, he was the only one in the oldest group who had the opportunity to acquire more advanced skills in the management of money as a result of his employment situation and access to community-based daily living and leisure activities.

Total scores for the 28 money tendering items were correlated with PPVT–R and WDRT age equivalent scores. A moderate level of association between receptive language (PPVT–R) and money tendering scores (r=.48) was found. There was a higher degree of association between reading (WDRT) and money scores (r=.68). This latter result could be explained by notes made by the interviewer during testing to the effect that many participants appeared to 'read' the value of the notes and coins presented to them. For this group, reading skills contributed to success in tasks involving money.

Interview questions probing participants' everyday use of money revealed that all but three could purchase small items such as a drink or pay a bus fare. One of this less competent group had lived in residential care for a number of years and had few of the functional skills needed for independent living. However, another individual, who had been in residential care since birth, travelled independently to her job in a sheltered workshop and had some functional money skills. Five of the participants were reported to 'budget their own money'; these skills generally involved allocating small sums for daily needs. One independent 19-year-old was reported to buy her own clothes.

When asked about their concerns for the future, only eight parents mentioned the management of money. Two of these parents had daughters who performed very poorly in the tendering tasks and both young women seemed to have had little opportunity, or encouragement, to acquire and use these skills.

Number skills

Only six of the participants could do all the simple addition sums correctly and one other made a single error. All were from integrated school situations. Two others did three of the sums correctly, both from special school backgrounds, one using her fingers and the other pointing to his head and saying 'Just think about it' in response to a query about how he calculated the answers. Half of the group did not attempt the number tasks, though three (from integrated settings) could do the sums using a calculator. There were no differences in terms of gender. In terms of age, the middle age group was most successful. The oldest group could not do these tasks.

The ease with which the addition sums were completed by CW, who had also completed all the money-tendering tasks successfully, drew the attention of the interviewer. Probing further, it became evident that the young woman was equally competent in subtraction, multiplication and division. From the age of three, she had attended a special school but at age 12 had moved to the local parochial school with her sisters. Here she was placed in a regular class where the teachers gave her activities appropriate for her level. Her family was aware that she was good at mathematics and encouraged her. She had a bank account and used a cash card. At the time of the interview, she was not working, but regularly accompanied her mother to a local club where they played in a bowling team and the girl kept score. Her exceptional number skills seemed to have resulted from positive expectations about her capacity to learn, coupled with opportunities to acquire competency in basic operations, and to use these skills in a meaningful context (e.g. bowling). This success can be contrasted with the lack of skills demonstrated by a 21-year-old male who could not do any of the simple addition sums and completed only the identification component of the money management task. At age 5 years, he had been noteworthy in his early intervention class for his competence in simple addition. From grade 5, he had attended a segregated school and at the time of the interview was working in a subsidized, but integrated workplace program. His mother reported that her son had no money skills, no cash card and no cheque book. She gave him money for outings. As with many others in the study, this young man had not maintained his early competence in numeracy and had not acquired appropriate skills for managing money in daily living.

Discussion

In summary, data presented here showed that the young adults who participated in the study could read digital time displays correctly, but had some difficulty with analogue displays. Almost all could recognize the value of coins and notes. Most could identify the cost of items from an advertisement, but only a quarter of the group could indicate the notes and/or coins needed to purchase an item. A slightly higher number stated that they would expect change, but these responses may not have been based on real understanding of the task. As noted earlier, only one participant was able to correctly calculate the amount of change that should be received and she clearly understood basic number concepts. There was no real difference between males and females in the number tasks, but in tendering money, the males tended to do better. In terms of age, the 21- to 24-year-old group did better than the 18- to 20-year-olds and both groups were more successful than the five oldest participants. There was a tendency for participants from integrated school backgrounds to do better on both number and money tendering tasks than those from special schools.

Clearly then, some young people with Down syndrome can acquire basic competence in functional number and money management skills. The skills displayed by CW, in particular, exemplify this finding. Three factors appeared to have contributed to her success: opportunity to learn, expectations of success and ongoing meaningful practice. These are key factors for people with Down syndrome and other types of intellectual disability who need to acquire basic numeracy and money management skills for independent or semi-independent living.

Undoubtedly, age and the type of school attended had an impact on the development of number and, more particularly money management skills in the young adults in the sample. In relation to age, it was evident that those born after the introduction of improved services for people with disabilities were more numerate than those born earlier. The consistently higher mean scores of the middle age group, when compared with the mean scores of younger participants, may have been an artefact of the sample. Another possible reason for this result lies with the higher expectations and increased opportunities to learn experienced by those born in the 1970s and later, following changes in the curriculum of special schools and increasing integration of children with Down syndrome into regular schools. However, it was also evident that, within the group born after 1970, those who were older (21-24 years of age) were more competent than the younger group (18-20 years of age). This finding may reflect the generally slower, but continuing, development of cognitive skills in young people with Down syndrome through adolescence and beyond. This issue was raised by Rynders (1999) and was demonstrated by Bashash (1997) who found that with increasing age, coupled with the opportunity to learn, students with moderate intellectual disabilities, including those with Down syndrome, continued to acquire higher levels of competence in number related skills.

Delays in finding a suitable job may have also led to additional time being spent at school or in school-related activities at Technical and Further Education (TAFE) colleges for the younger group of students. In fact, all participants in the middle age-group were involved in open or supported employment, or in a sheltered workshop, either full- or part-time, where they had opportunities to earn and handle money. In contrast, those aged 18-20 years were still mainly at school, in work experience placements or under-taking training in a TAFE college, with only small numbers involved in open and supported employment or a sheltered workshop. Opportunity to practise skills is crucial if they are to be retained. Participants were most competent at those numeracy skills that were clearly related to everyday activities, such as recognition of prices and digital time.

Those individuals who had received their education in an integrated setting generally did better on the assessment tasks than those who had a segregated background. Similar results were evident in the reading test scores reported in Bochner et al. (in press), with the integrated group scoring higher on the WDRT at both the youngest and middle age levels. Interestingly, this pattern was not evident in the PPVT-R scores reported by Bochner et al., where the youngest segregated group did better than the youngest integrated group, suggesting that type of school may have a greater impact on school-related achievement (i.e. reading and mathematics) than on the more generic receptive language skills assessed by the PPVT-R.

Conclusion

Data reported here suggest that at least some individuals with Down syndrome can acquire basic number skills and functional money management skills that are not simply learned by rote but reflect real understanding of underlying concepts. Yet not all such young people have the opportunity to acquire these skills, either at school or at home. Efforts need to be made to identify the basic number and money skills needed to function within the community. Appropriate training programs should be provided from an early age and continued until well into the post-school years. Parents and carers must be convinced that young people with Down syndrome should not only be given the opportunity to acquire these skills, but that they need to use them in meaningful contexts and to practise the skills regularly.

References

Baroody AJ (1986) Basic counting principles used by mentally retarded children. Journal of Research in Mathematics Education 17: 382-9.

Baroody AJ (1988) Number-comparison learning by children classified as mentally retarded. American Journal on Mental Retardation 92: 461-71.

Baroody AJ (1995) The role of number-after rule in the invention of computational short-cuts. Cognition and Instruction 13: 189-219.

Baroody AJ, Snyder P (1983) A cognitive analysis of basic arithmetic abilities of TMR children. Education and Training of the Mentally Retarded 18: 253-9.

Bashash L (1997) Counting skills and concepts of number in children with moderate intellectual disabilities. Unpublished doctoral dissertation, Macquarie University, Sydney, Australia.

Bashash L, Outhred L (1996) Number comparison skills of children with moderate intellectual disabilities. In Clarkson PC (Ed) Proceedings of the 19th Annual Conference of the Mathematics Education Research Group of Australasia. Melbourne: Mathematics Education Research Group of Australasia. pp 72-9.

Berry P, Groenweg G, Gibson D, Brown RI (1984) Mental development of adults with Down Syndrome. American Journal of Mental Deficiency 89: 252-6.

Bochner S, Outhred L, Pieterse M (in press). Functional literacy skills in young adults with Down syndrome. International Journal of Developmental Disabilities.

Carr J (1995) Down's Syndrome: Children Growing Up. Cambridge: Cambridge University Press.

Caycho L, Gunn P, Siegal M (1991) Counting by children with Down Syndrome. American Journal on Mental Retardation 95: 575-83.

Center Y, Ferguson C, Ward J (1988) The Integration of Children with Disabilities into Regular Classrooms (Mainstreaming): A Naturalistic Study. Stage 1 Report. Sydney: Macquarie University.

Cornwell AC (1974) Development of language, abstraction and concept formation in home-reared children with Down's syndrome (mongolism). American Journal of Mental Deficiency 74: 179-90.

Dunn LM, Dunn LM (1981) Peabody Picture Vocabulary Test - Revised. Circle Pines, MN: American Guidance Services.

Dunn LM, Markwardt F (1970) Peabody Individual Achievement Test. Circle Pines, MN: American Guidance Services.

Fuson KC (1988) Children's Counting and Concepts of Number. New York: Springer-Verlag.

Gelman R (1982) Basic numerical abilities. In Sternberg RJ (Ed) Advances in the Psychology of Intelligence: Vol 1. Hillsdale, NJ: Erlbaum. pp 181-205.

Gelman R, Cohen M (1988) Qualitative differences in the way Down syndrome and normal children solve a novel counting task. In Nadel L (Ed) The Psychobiology of Down Syndrome. London: MIT Press. pp 51-100.

Gelman R, Gallistel CR (1978) The Child's Understanding of Number. Cambridge, MA: Harvard University Press.

Pieterse M (1988) The Down syndrome program at Macquarie University: a model early intervention program. In Pieterse M, Bochner S, Bettison S (Eds) Early Intervention for Children with Disabilities: The Australian Experience. Sydney: Macquarie University. pp 81-96.

Pieterse M, Bochner S, Bettison S (1988) Early Intervention for Children with Disabilities: The Australian Experience. Sydney: Macquarie University.

Pieterse M, Center Y (1984) The integration of eight Down's syndrome children into regular schools. Australian and New Zealand Journal of Developmental Disabilities 10: 11-20.

Rynders JE (1996) The school years: Becoming literate and socialized. In Rynders JE, Horrobin JM (Eds) Down Syndrome: Birth to Adulthood: Giving Families an EDGE. Denver: Love. pp 163-90.

Rynders JE (1999) Promoting the educational competence of students with DS. In Rondal J, Perera J, Nadel L (Eds) Down Syndrome: A Review of Current Knowledge. London: Whurr. pp 64-78.

Rynders JE, Horrobin JM (1996) Down Syndrome - Birth to Adulthood: Giving Families an EDGE. Denver: Love.

Smith G, Spiker D, Peterson C, Ciccetti D, Justine P (1984) Use of megadoses of vitamins with minerals in Down Syndrome. Journal of Pediatrics 105: 228-34.

Steffe LP, von Glasersfeld E, Richards E, Cobb P (1983) Children's Counting Types: Philosophy, Theory and Application. New York: Praeger Scientific.

Waddington NJ (1988) Waddington Diagnostic Reading and Spelling Test: A Book of Tests and Diagnostic Procedures for Children with Learning Difficulties. Ingle Farm, SA: Waddington Educational Resources.

SECTION 5
ADULT LIFE

Introduction

Anne Jobling and Monica Cuskelly have collected information from a large number of adults with Down syndrome. This study has the largest number of participants of any study of its kind and so provides much useful information about the lives of adults. Social, cultural, and political differences between countries mean, however, that their results should be treated cautiously by those from other countries and studies of adult life are to be encouraged in other places. Of note is the continuing reliance of the adults with Down syndrome on parental support for access to the life of their community. This suggests that community services are inadequate for this age group and also raises the issue of preparation for independent living. Several authors of previous chapters have discussed the need for a greater emphasis on the development of self-regulatory skills (see, for example, Glenn and Cunningham, and Giorcelli) in young people with Down syndrome.

The group of researchers from Flinders University (Verity Bottroff, Roy Brown, Eddie Bullitis, Vicky Duffield, John Grantley, Margaret Kyrkou and Judy Thornley) have written about the quality of life of adults with Down syndrome and provided some markers that assist us to determine if individuals are enjoying a reasonable quality of life. The studies briefly described in their chapter cover a wide range of life aspects but all share the common thread of enlarging our understanding of the quality of life of those with Down syndrome. Quality of life researchers have contributed substantially to our recognition of the negative impact of some of the practices common in services for, and research about, individuals with an intellectual disability. This chapter, therefore, resonates with the thrust apparent in the opening chapter of this book, by Jan Gothard, of encouraging individuals with Down syndrome to be allowed to speak for themselves whenever possible. The issue of quality of life is also indirectly addressed by Roy McConkey in his chapter on developing services for those with a disability in the third world. The chapter by Bottroff and colleagues should persuade all researchers to consider the role they are allowing those with Down syndrome to play in the research process and may even encourage some to work collaboratively with those with Down syndrome.

Clearly, engagement in the workforce is one criterion for quality of life for an adult. Anna Contardi describes a programme that has been running in Italy for several years that aims to assist young adults with Down syndrome

succeed in working independently in a service industry. She supplies a level
of detail that will be helpful to others interested in developing a similar
programme and provides a very encouraging progress report. Contardi
argues that the success of the programme relies on a certain level of skill and
self-awareness on the part of the young person with Down syndrome and on
the right organizational structure. All of these she sees as being open to influence and therefore she reasons that the success she reports need not be an
isolated occurrence but could become widespread.

CHAPTER 9

Life styles of adults with Down syndrome living at home

ANNE JOBLING AND MONICA CUSKELLY

Introduction

The life circumstances of persons with intellectual disabilities have changed markedly over the last 15 years (Brown, 1995). Now, with deinstitutionalization, improved health care, increased services and community participation, individuals with intellectual disabilities enjoy extended life opportunities that were once denied them. These life opportunities present individuals with many more challenging life events than experienced by those of previous decades. Moreover, education programs available from birth into adulthood (i.e. 18 years of age) have provided many opportunities for individuals with intellectual disability to gain skills. For some years, a common focus of the majority of secondary school programs for those with intellectual disability has been to provide curricula aimed at developing skills that will enable a successful transition from school to community. These skills are seen to be those that relate to independence, self-help, work experience and training, and leisure. The transition curriculum has now replaced the traditional school content related to academic skills. Transition programming (see Riches, 1996, for a description of the various types) is seen as an essential component in the development of quality of life outcomes for young people with intellectual disability as they leave school and move towards life in the community. In Queensland, where the study reported below was conducted, transition programs now form the basis of secondary education for most adolescents with Down syndrome.

Clearly, such a change of educational practice should be subject to rigorous evaluation; however, to date, no data reporting on this curriculum change are available. Furthermore, there is limited information about the life styles of individuals with Down syndrome post-school. While there have been several investigations of the life circumstances of adults with intellectual disability, including those with Down syndrome, these have primarily focused on adults of 50 years and over (e.g. Ashman, Suttie and Bramley, 1993; Bigby, 1997, 1998; Buys and Rushworth, 1997). Scant attention has been paid to investigating the lives of young adults, that is, the time between the young adults leaving secondary school transition programs and their senior years.

Several factors may have contributed to this. In past years, there was a common belief that the life expectancy of children with Down syndrome would not extend beyond 12 years, but by the 1980s it was considered that almost half of the population born with Down syndrome would survive to age 60 (Carr, 1995). In addition, research demonstrated a higher than normal incidence of dementia in older individuals with intellectual disability, especially those with Down syndrome (Janicki and Dalton, 2000). The recognition of the extension of life expectancy, potential medical concerns plus the accompanying move from institutions into the community, resulted in a strong focus on older adults with Down syndrome, to the relative neglect of younger adults.

This younger group seems to be invisible to researchers possibly because most adults continue to live at home with their families after leaving school and thus do not place great demands on service providers. For example, Fujiura (1998) produced demographic data in the USA on individuals with intellectual disability and found that the vast majority of individuals lived in the family residence and were supported by parents, relatives or other carers. The majority of persons with disabilities in Queensland (86 per cent) live at home, and family members are the primary providers of assistance.

Other researchers have found that the family plays a major role in the life of the adult with intellectual disability (Carr, 1995; Essex, Seltzer and Krauss, 1999; Fujiura, 1998; Seltzer, 1992; Seltzer and Krauss, 1994). As Fujiura stated: '. . . the family is fundamentally important to the American system of care' (1998: 234). Seltzer (1992) concurred with this view, arguing that it is only when ageing parents can no longer cope or when the effects of ageing further handicap the person with an intellectual disability that this invisible population becomes evident.

Some information about life post-school for individuals with Down syndrome is available. There are several biographical works which deal with this life stage (e.g. Hunt, 1967; Kingsley and Levitz, 1994; Moody and Moody, 1986). A few reports have been published using American data (Nagel and Rosenthal, 1995; Rynders and Horrobin, 1996), and Carr (1995) using information collected in Britain, also reported on patterns of daytime occupations post-school. All of these studies had small numbers of participants.

Carr (1995) followed up a sample of 35 young adults with Down syndrome aged 21 years. Fifteen per cent of the group were at home full time. She reported that only 10 per cent of her sample worked (all were part time) and this work was on farms or in family businesses, with one individual working in hairdressing. The remaining 75 per cent attended local day centres where a variety of activities from crafts and cooking to work training were undertaken. Most could not get to work independently and required special transport arrangements. Questions about recreational activities at home revealed that books (78 per cent), drawing (49 per cent), and board games (39 per cent) were popular. Listening to music (93 per cent) and television watching (90 per cent) were daily activities. Sixty-one per cent played one or more sports with 58 per cent swimming at least weekly, table tennis was popular with 35 per cent of the young people, and 66 per cent of the group went to dances or leisure clubs enjoyed by their parents.

The young adults made a contribution to the household with 93 per cent doing some housework and a smaller proportion undertaking cooking. However, parents played a major role in facilitating community involvement. Sixty-six per cent of the adults went shopping with their parents and 53 per cent took their holidays accompanied by parent/s. Carr noted that ability alone was not sufficient to guarantee that the young adult would reach a level of independence, but that urban and rural factors as well as mothers' beliefs influenced the adults' life style.

The 15 young men aged 25 years who participated in the 'EDGE' project (Rynders and Horrobin, 1996) appeared to have opportunities to engage more fully in community life. These young people had an age appropriate interest in popular culture, all participated in sports through Special Olympics, and the males followed a sporting team. All young adults worked or were attending job preparation programs.

In studies reporting on community participation for people with Down syndrome, Scouts, tertiary schooling, sports, religious activities, jobs, and travel were listed as some of their out of school activities (Nagel and Rosenthal, 1995; Wehman, 1995). Wehman (1995) reported that there were now improved employment opportunities which had moved beyond sheltered employment for these young people.

Now, it would seem that individuals with Down syndrome aspire to be part of the community: 'Being part of the community is important for all people whether they have Down syndrome or not – I live an exciting and happy life' (Christopher Burke, cited in Nagel and Rosenthal, 1995: ix); and that individuals with Down syndrome 'are no longer considered "eternal children" who will spend the rest of their lives within our protective embrace or the safety of a sheltered workshop' (Kingsley and Kingsley, cited in Pueschel and Sustrova, 1997: 1). Little is known, however, about the realization of these aspirations in their lives after school.

The study reported here aimed to provide preliminary data about various aspects of life style in a sample of adults with Down syndrome who lived at home with their families in Queensland, Australia. The participants lived in metropolitan, regional and country areas. No Australian study has previously reported this information, and it may be inappropriate to base conclusions on the results of studies with small numbers from other countries.

Data collection

A specifically designed life style questionnaire was mailed to 400 families who had an adult member (18 years and over) with Down syndrome. Data were obtained on 173 adults who lived in the family home and, of these, 110 adults aged 19 to 45 years (mean age 27.68 years, SD 7.11) were selected for analysis. The other 63 were still attending school at 18 years, were retired or in poor health. The majority of family respondents were mothers of the adult with Down syndrome (66 per cent). Others who completed the questionnaire were family members such as fathers and siblings.

The questionnaire focused on five aspects of adult life: employment, leisure activities, post-school courses, reading, and religious observance. The questionnaire asked the respondents to provide information about the type of activity, average hours of engagement per week, form of travel taken to the activity, individual choices about activity type, and the support necessary for the individual to participate. Questions about favourite pastimes, family chores, friendships and wages were also included.

Results

There were no significant differences between the responses of the metropolitan, regional or country participants so the data were combined for analysis. This was in contrast to Carr's (1995) data that found urban and rural factors influenced life style opportunities.

Employment

It was reported that 72 (41 males) individuals (65 per cent) were employed and of these 39 lived in Brisbane, the major city in Queensland. The main types of work in which the adults with Down syndrome engaged were packing, collating and associated mailroom work, although some respondents were not exactly clear about the type of work the person with Down syndrome undertook. Eight adults were employed doing outdoor work. Sheltered workshops (n=47) were the primary location of work, 13 adults were employed in private enterprise, and 12 others had a variety of work with employment services. Forty-eight adults were paid for their work and the type of payment was primarily a wage plus pension (*n*=44). Most of the young adults (*n*=51) worked between 20 to 40 hours per week and others worked less than 10 hours. These employment opportunities were mainly accessed through employment support agencies and school transitional work experience programs.

Leisure activities

Seven leisure activities: the Arts, Sports, Crafts, Movies, Shopping, Holidays, and Day outings or trips were specifically chosen for the questionnaire from various leisure inventories. They were considered representative of the community leisure interests of adults with intellectual disability. The types of activities, frequency of participation, where and how organized, and with whom they undertook the activity are shown in Table 9.1. Many individuals participated in a number of leisure pursuits.

In addition, respondents were asked to nominate the adults' favourite activities (more than one activity could be nominated). Over 20 activities were included in this list, with concerts featuring music groups, plays and

Table 9.1 Participation in Leisure Activities

Activity	Main types	How often	Who organizes	Attends with
Arts (*n* = 76)	Dancing Music Drama	Weekly or monthly	Agency	Agency
Crafts (*n* = 35)	Various	Weekly	Agency	Agency
Holidays (*n* = 92)	Family	Annual or twice yearly	Parent	Parent
Day out (*n* = 89)	14 different types reported	Weekly or fortnightly	Parent	Parent/ agency
Movies (*n* = 82)	Various Action movies most popular	Monthly	Parent	Parent
Shopping (*n* = 86)	Personal items and food (mostly accompanied)	Weekly	Parent	Parent
Sports (*n* = 73)	Various	Weekly	Parent/ agency	Club/ agency

musical comedy performances (63 per cent), television and videos (43 per cent), sports participation (43 per cent) and outings which included shopping, visits and dining out with family (27 per cent) being the most frequent responses. A wide range of television programmes were watched but the favourites were soaps/sitcoms, and musical variety programmes, and these were mainly watched alone (only 18 respondents recorded that the adult with Down syndrome watched with others). The time spent watching television through the week ranged from under 10 hours (20 per cent), 10 to 21 hours (52 per cent) and over 21 hours (28 per cent) with one report of 44 hours of television watching per week.

Religious observance

Involvement in religious activities was reported for 51 adults (27 males). Their attendance was usually weekly or fortnightly at church services with the family or a friendship club. This observance was primarily organized by the family and took place locally.

Post-school study courses

More than half of the adults (*n*=59, 24 males) were undertaking some course of further study. These were basically undertaken to improve skills and five of the adults had been responsible for the decision to attend further training. The courses included educational programs (literacy and numeracy; *n*=29); programs provided by Activity Therapy Centres which focused on life skills training (*n*=19); work training programs (*n*=7) and training in the performing arts (*n*=2). Two individuals were in unspecified programs. Attendance at these courses varied from daily to twice a week and the length of involvement was from six weeks to 12 months. Some adults took more than one course over the year. The courses were mainly taken in an educational or agency facility, with a teacher or agency representative, and attendance was organized by a parent or the agency.

Reading

Reading was reported as an activity for 54 (26 males) of the adults in the study. It was either a daily or weekly activity and mainly involved reading newspapers and magazines (*n*=38). Usually the reading took place at home (*n*=42) with virtually no use of public libraries. Those questions that attempted to gain information about with whom the adult read or when their interest in reading developed were poorly answered, but 47 adults chose their own material to read, ten of these with some help.

Friendships

Although some respondents were not able to answer the questions about friendships, stating they did not know, it was reported that most adults had friends (83 per cent), of whom 30 per cent were within the family. Friendships were primarily linked to the work place, with 36 adults reported to have friends at work. Participation in recreational activities provided another avenue for the development of friends. Some had a boy/girl friend relationship, some had imaginary friends and a few had a pen friend.

Helping at home

Most of the adults helped daily with chores in the home and were considered to be either very good (49 per cent) or satisfactory (45 per cent) at the tasks they undertook. The tasks ranged from being responsible for self and others to inside and outside household chores. Responsibility for self (62 per cent: dressing, hygiene and room tidying) and household tasks (81 per cent) were the most frequent tasks executed by the adults with Down syndrome.

Life style difference between younger and older persons with Down syndrome

In order to examine whether there were life style differences in this living at home sample due to age, two age groups were identified initially (see below) then persons within these age groups were randomly selected for the comparison. One group (n=6.6) represented a younger age group (19 to 22 years), while the other (n=16) represented an older age group (30 to 42 years). The younger group were born and grew up during a period of time when early intervention, inclusive schooling and transitional planning and programs were regular features of the education for children with Down syndrome in Queensland, while the older group did not have these initiatives available to them.

Employment opportunities were comparable for both groups with the sheltered workshop being the main work place. Post-school study courses were undertaken more often by the younger group and these related to literacy, preparation for more inclusive styles of employment, and the performing arts (music and drama). Only one of the older age group (aged 39 years) was reported to have attended a course that was intended to provide literacy and other skill development. Both groups had friends and these were primarily seen at work. Both groups had imaginary friends who were sometimes a television character or a pop-star. As with the larger data set, agencies and families played a dominant role in organizing and attending activities with the adult with Down syndrome, irrespective of age group. Sports, day outings and activities associated with the arts were primarily initiated by the family but were organized and supervised by agencies, while movies, holidays, church, shopping and reading were activities undertaken within the family. This was true for both age groups; however, there was more ability to travel independently in the younger age group. Favourite activities across the groups were similar, with sports, listening to music and watching television being the most popular.

Clearly, this comparison must be treated cautiously as the numbers are so small. However, it does indicate that some changes are occurring in the lives of adults with Down syndrome, so studies conducted some years ago may not be informative about the current situation.

Discussion

Work was the main activity outside the home for these adults with Down syndrome. There were some successful placements by community employment agencies but the main avenue for employment remained the sheltered workshop, and agency help when seeking a job was found to be essential. These results are in contrast to those of Carr (1995), who reported that only 10 per cent of her sample worked, and are slightly higher than those of Neumayer and Bleasdale (1996), who reported that 50 per cent of their sample worked in sheltered workshops. Reid and Hitchcock (1996) also reported limited participation in the community via work, with the majority of their participants spending their days in a segregated workshop or activity centre. There was little to support Wehman's (1995) suggestion that work options had moved beyond the sheltered workshop. The type of payment received by the adults with Down syndrome in the study reported here reflects the Australian Social Services System where wages are adjusted to retain other benefits such as a health card or transport allowances. For the family, anxieties can result if these benefits are lost. The types of work and pay were similar to those reported in a small New Zealand study by Reid and Bray (1997).

Leisure activities were varied, although families and agencies once again assumed the major role in facilitating these activities and accompanying the adult to the activities. This was in comparison to Neumayer and Bleasdale's (1996) sample where 67 per cent were considered to be independent in pursuing their leisure activities. It was also noted that the adult's choice of a favourite activity was often at home (television, videos and music CDs) or related to family activity (outings) and, in the case of television, the activity was mostly solitary. These were also the activities they enjoyed most in Neumayer and Bleasdale's (1996) life preferences survey. Sports participation was an exception to this trend of preferring home activities, similar to Carr (1995) who reported sport participation for 80 per cent of her sample. The arts was one activity where involvement was high, albeit with the ever-present support of an agency. This was in contrast to findings by Brown (1994) where spectator and low activity interests seem to be predominant.

In Queensland, although services have been slow to develop, it is encouraging to note that families, knowing their adult child's interest in these activities, were able to assist them to access agencies that could enable them to participate. Agencies for sports (Q-RAPID and Special Olympics) and the arts (Access Arts and D'Arts) have provided and continue to provide opportunities in community based programs. These organizations have often led the way in providing inclusive opportunities in community managed and organized activities such as sport (Jobling, 1999), but these results indicate more needs to be done to develop choice and independence.

Few socializing opportunities were reported with friends in clubs or on outings, and attendance at church activities was a family occasion. Similar to Bigby (1997) – with an older population – the family network played a key socializing role. Bigby noted that it was important to recognize that social networks beyond the family tended to be related to specific programs (for example a day centre or work), so changes in attendance must be carefully planned and well-managed. Television, videos and music CDs provide many entertaining and educational benefits for the adult, but they can add to their isolation from the community and also from their family. Lack of independence in travelling limits opportunities, and friendships which are restricted to work or within the family could also add to this isolation, especially as individuals retire from work.

Post-school educational opportunities were limited. For these adult learners, continuity of learning opportunities is important (Moni and Jobling, 2000), but as the questions related to the length of involvement were poorly answered, it was difficult to ascertain continuity. As Fowler, Doherty and Boynton (1995) also noted with regard to literacy, most adults had not progressed. Fowler et al. hypothesized that many adults had not received the appropriate instruction, a hypothesis that is confirmed within the Queensland context. Also it would seem that although Fowler and others have suggested that the after school years may in fact be an optimal time to introduce reading and other literacy activities, facilitation and support for such activities was limited. Although further education courses of six to ten weeks are an accepted part of transitional programs, it could be suggested that there is a need to offer long-term and continuing options at varying entry levels. In this study, reading was primarily a home activity and there was limited use of public facilities, even although Queensland has good local and visiting mobile libraries.

The central, and often solitary, role of the family in facilitating the life style of their adult with Down syndrome was evident across all aspects of the study. As also shown by Fujiura (1998) and Smith (1997), families, particularly mothers, bear a heavy duty of care either themselves or in combination with an agency. Agency support was essential to families in this study; however, funding for such support is often precarious (Sheppardson, 1992, cited in Carr, 1995). The responsibility that many parents take in caring for their adult child with disabilities can have profound implications for other aspects of their lives (Einam and Cuskelly, in preparation; Harland and Cuskelly, 2000).

The high level of family management and care of adults with Down syndrome is of concern as the normative life stages through which families progress as their children grow up tend to be disrupted when an adult family member requires the level of continual support indicated by these data. Mothers were the main respondents and this is not surprising as mothers are seen as the prime managers of the educational, social, domestic and vocational needs of their child or adult with a lifelong intellectual disability (Harland and Cuskelly, 2000; Essex et al., 1999). In this study, parent/s continued to have a high level of involvement with organizing activities such as holidays, day outings, movie-going, shopping, sports participation and church activities, and were the most frequent accompanying person for holidays, days out, movies and shopping. As stated by Carr (1995), it seemed for these families of an adult with Down syndrome the normative stages were altered. This high level of involvement may have been exacerbated by the low levels of independence reported in the adult person with Down syndrome, in both the organization of and attendance at an activity.

Family involvement in the planning and implementation of life's activities placed demands on parents some decades beyond normal parenting responsibilities, an outcome also reported by Essex et al. (1999). This dependence on parents may have implications for the adult with Down syndrome as well as the parents. Collacott and Cooper (1997) found a decline in language and other adaptive behaviour scores in adults with Down syndrome living at home. They suggested that these declines may have their origin in the increasing dependence of the adult with Down syndrome on a parent who is ageing, combined with their isolated life style.

Although it is acknowledged that there are limitations with the voluntary way in which these data were collected, they present the life circumstances of a large sample of individuals with Down syndrome, living at home. Clearly, the lives of the individuals represented here are restricted in many ways with relatively little involvement in the wider community and an unacceptable reliance on their parents for practical and social support. As individuals with Down syndrome now live longer, the demands on parents will continue, unless the unmet needs of this heretofore invisible group are recognized.

Recent research has challenged the view that the burden of care experienced by elderly parents is necessarily viewed by them as negative (Krauss and Seltzer, 1995) and some benefits to parents have been identified (Seltzer and Krauss, 1993). Indeed there is evidence that some adults with intellectual impairment take a broader role in the family and extend their skills as their parents age (Krauss and Seltzer, 1998). It is important to ensure, however, that these studies are not used to undermine the push for appropriate services for adults with an intellectual impairment, and that both individuals with Down syndrome and their families have choices about the level of support that parents continue to provide.

References

Ashman AF, Suttie J, Bramley J (1993) Older Australians with an Intellectual Disability. Brisbane: The University of Queensland, Fred and Eleanor Schonell Special Educational Research Centre.

Bigby C (1997) Later life for adults with intellectual disability: a time of opportunity and vulnerability. Journal of Intellectual and Developmental Disability 22: 97–108.

Bigby C (1998) Shifting responsibilities: the pattern of formal service use by older people with intellectual disability in Victoria. Journal of Intellectual and Developmental Disability 23: 229–43.

Brown RI (1994) Down syndrome and quality of life: some challenges for future practice. Down's Syndrome Research and Practice 2: 19–30.

Brown RI (1995) Quality of Life for People with Disabilities. Cheltenham: Stanley Thornes.

Buys LR, Rushworth JS (1997) Community services available to older adults with intellectual disabilities. Journal of Intellectual and Developmental Disability 22: 27–37.

Carr J (1995) Down's Syndrome: Children Growing Up. London: Cambridge University Press.

Collacott RA, Cooper SA (1997) Five year follow-up study of adaptive behaviour in adults with Down Syndrome. Journal of Intellectual and Developmental Disability 22: 187–97.

Disability: A Queensland Profile (1999) Brisbane: Queensland Government.

Einam M, Cuskelly M (in preparation) Paid employment of mothers and fathers of an adult child with multiple disabilities. Available from M Cuskelly.

Essex EL, Seltzer MM, Krauss MW (1999) Differences in coping effectiveness and well-being among aging mothers and fathers of adults with mental retardation. American Journal on Mental Retardation 104: 545–63.

Fowler A, Doherty BJ, Boynton L (1995) Basis of reading skill in young adults with Down syndrome. In Nagel L, Rosenthal D (Eds) Down Syndrome: Living and Learning in the Community. New York: Wiley-Liss. pp 182–96.

Fujiura GT (1998) Demography of family households. American Journal on Mental Retardation 103: 225–35.

Harland P, Cuskelly M (2000) The responsibilities of adult siblings of adults with dual sensory impairments. International Journal of Disability, Development and Education 47: 293–307.

Hunt N (1967) The World of Nigel Hunt: The Diary of a Mongoloid Youth. Beaconsfield: Darwen Finlayson.

Janicki MP, Dalton AJ (2000) Prevalence of dementia and impact on intellectual disability services. Mental Retardation 38: 276–88.

Jobling A (1999) Queensland. In Lockwood R, Lockwood A (Eds) Recreation and Disability in Australia. Perth, Australia: DUIT Multimedia. pp 214–28.

Kingsley J, Levitz M (1994) Count Us In: Growing up with Down Syndrome. New York: Harcourt Brace.

Krauss MW, Seltzer MM (1995) Long-term caring: family experiences over the life course. In Nagel L, Rosenthal D (Eds) Down Syndrome: Living and Learning in the Community. New York: Wiley-Liss. pp 91–8.

Krauss MW, Seltzer MM (1998) Life course perspectives in mental retardation research: the case of family caregiving. In Burack LJA, Hodapp RM, Zigler E (Eds) Handbook of Mental Retardation and Development. Cambridge: Cambridge University Press. pp 504–20.

Moni K, Jobling A (2000) LATCH-ON: A program to develop literacy in young adults with Down syndrome. Journal of Adolescent and Adult Literacy 44: 40–9.

Moody P, Moody R (1986) Half left. Oslo, Norway: Dreyers Forlag.

Nagel L, Rosenthal D (1995) Down Syndrome: Living and Learning in the Community. New York: Wiley-Liss.

Neumayer R, Bleasdale M (1996) Personal lifestyle preferences of people with intellectual disability. Journal of Intellectual and Developmental Disability 21: 91–114.

Pueschel SM, Sustrova M (1997) Adolescents with Down Syndrome. Baltimore: Paul H. Brookes.

Reid PM, Bray A (1997) Paid work and intellectual disability. Journal of Intellectual and Developmental Disability 22: 87–96.

Reid PM, Hitchcock D (1996) Continuing education and intellectual disability. In Bennie G (Ed) Supported Employment in New Zealand. Levin, New Zealand: Network Publications.

Riches V (1996) A review of transition from school to community for students with disabilities in NSW Australia. Journal of Intellectual and Developmental Disability 21: 71–88.

Rynders JE, Horrobin JM (1996) Down Syndrome: Birth to Adulthood – Giving Families an EDGE. London: Love Publishing Company.

Seltzer MM (1992) Family caregiving across the full life span. In L Rowitz (Ed) Mental Retardation in the Year 2000. New York: Springer-Verlag. pp 85–100.

Seltzer MM, Krauss MW (1993) Current well-being and future plans of older caregiving mothers. Irish Journal of Psychology 14: 47–64.

Seltzer MM, Krauss MW (1994) Aging parents with resident adult children: the impact of lifelong caring. In Seltzer MM, Krauss MW, Janicki MP (Eds) Lifespan Course Perspectives on Adulthood and Old Age. Washington, DC: American Association on Mental Retardation. pp 3–18.

Smith GC (1997) Ageing families of adults with mental retardation: patterns and correlates of service use, needs and knowledge. American Journal on Mental Retardation 102: 13–26.

Wehman P (1995) Supported employment for people with disabilities: what progress has been made? In Nagel L, Rosenthal D (Eds) Down Syndrome: Living and Learning in the Community. New York: Wiley-Liss. pp 263–75.

CHAPTER 10
Some studies involving individuals with Down syndrome and their relevance to a quality of life model

VERITY BOTTROFF, ROY BROWN, EDDIE BULLITIS, VICKY DUFFIELD, JOHN GRANTLEY, MARGARET KYRKOU AND JUDY THORNLEY

The following chapter presents a series of studies being undertaken in the School of Special Education and Disability Studies, at Flinders University in South Australia. The studies are only loosely connected but they share a common focus on aspects of the quality of life of individuals with Down syndrome. Although this is not the place to go into any depth explaining the construct of quality of life (for detailed discussion, see Brown, 1997) it is relevant to point out some of its underlying features. In this context it is essentially a social and psychological concept. It has both quantitative and qualitative dimensions and is about family and individual stories and narratives as well as numerical information about health and performance (Renwick and Brown, 1996).

One of its major attributes is the importance placed on personal perception by the individual with a disability, regardless of level of knowledge, performance, or language. That is, statements made by the individual, whether verbal or nonverbal, are acknowledged and used as central components in understanding behaviours. This is critical when considering the lives of those with Down syndrome since parental and professional opinions often over-ride the views and choices of persons with a disability. Indeed, the individual views of persons with Down syndrome may be ignored, despite the fact that it has been clearly shown that individuals' perceptions, i.e. what they think, feel and choose, frequently determine their behaviour. The extent to which an individual's views are acknowledged is believed to influence self-image, ability to control the environment and to assist individuals develop an internal locus of control (see IASSID, 2000: Report on Quality of Life). Proxy statements on behalf of the individual are seen as suspect and often do not

121

represent the views of the individual (Cummins, 1997). This does not deny the importance of parental or professional opinion but it must be recognized that these are not substitutes for the individual's own views. From a quality of life perspective, the concern is not whether the views of the individual with a disability are correct or incorrect in terms of the objective situation, but that the thoughts of the individual are taken into account.

Quality of life is also about well-being in health, education, employment and engagement in the community, but it is primarily concerned with the whole individual and how she or he experiences life. This cannot be determined by any one science like medicine or psychology, or perhaps by science as a whole; it represents an expression of the individual within a family and has to be applied in an holistic manner. Science and technology may assist but can only be effective if they, in the end, are directed toward the overall well-being or satisfaction of the individual and family. Thus quality of life is multidisciplinary and holistic (i.e. it concerns the integrated aspects of life for the individual).

Quality of life also includes the concept of life span. What happens at any one point in time influences what happens later. Early development and experience help to determine later well-being and quality of life. This is particularly relevant to those with Down syndrome since such individuals' longevity is rapidly increasing, giving rise to new challenges for adult life. Needs and choices experienced by the individual are also critical, though they should be seen within a family context. Such concepts raise the importance of inclusive practices, since choices can be applied most effectively where there is involvement with non-disabled peers in a regular community. Thus the quality and range of experience at school, for example, is likely to influence employment opportunities and in turn the type of family life and eventual retirement experiences of each individual.

Another feature of such a quality of life model is that it encourages parents and professionals to look at differences amongst individuals and not simply respond to a diagnostic label. Indeed, research and practice from this perspective underscore individual variation and alert the reader to interpret information when interacting with an individual with Down syndrome.

Thus, quality of life is a sensitizing concept focusing attention on the individual's well-being and self-expression within the context of his or her environment. Adopting this perspective leads to changes in the focus of research and practice. In particular, much of the data from such research will come from the individuals themselves, either through verbal statements or through observation of individual behaviour, this latter method being used in cases where the person has little or no verbal behaviour. Any research will recognize that the choices and opinions of individuals with Down syndrome must be taken into account when designing studies.

The following studies look at some of these issues, and the reader is encouraged to see how each separate report relates to present and future activities that might represent development for specific individuals with Down syndrome. It is suggested the above comments be applied to see how quality of life issues were taken into account in each study. We would argue, however, that it is the integration of our understanding of the various aspects of the lives of those with Down syndrome that is often lacking in our society. The challenge is how to bring information surrounding these concepts together for the benefit of the individual and their family.

Study 1: Recognizing period pain: PMS in women with Down syndrome

(Primary reseacher: Margaret Kyrkou)

Initially called premenstrual tension (PMT) by Frank in 1931, premenstrual syndrome (PMS) is still a nebulous condition with no specific diagnostic tests. However, whether or not they have a disability, for many sufferers and their families and friends, it results in significant distress. PMS is defined as 'the presence of recurrent symptoms before menstruation with the complete absence of symptoms after menstruation' (Dalton and Holton, 1994). Symptoms that recur on and off throughout the menstrual cycle, even though they might be worse premenstrually, are not due to PMS. Although PMS was medically recognized in the 1930s, and over 350 clinical trials have been conducted since 1964, most professionals are only aware of a few of the 100 or more symptoms (Mortola, 1995). Theories of causation have abounded over the years, but none have been able to be proven. There is a growing suspicion that the premenstrual fall in progesterone is a significant factor in the causation of premenstrual symptoms.

As reported below, women with Down syndrome, and their families and carers, face an even greater challenge in recognizing PMS, as symptoms reported by women with Down syndrome, their families and carers, differ significantly from those described by women in the general population. The few brief references to PMS in books relating to disability do not allude to possible differences in the expression of the condition. The combination of professional ignorance about the breadth of symptomatology associated with PMS and lack of information specific to women with an intellectual disability mean that the diagnosis is likely to be disregarded in this group.

Issues in diagnosing the condition

Readers might question the need to diagnose such a nebulous condition, but it is important to recognize the true diagnosis in order to avoid inappropriate management:

- Behavioural symptoms may be diagnosed as being due to a psychiatric condition, and powerful medication prescribed. If the medication fails to control the behaviour, or the behaviour re-emerges after the premenstrual phase of that cycle has passed (the next premenstrual phase having begun), the dose of medication might be increased on the assumption that the previous dose was insufficient.
- Behavioural symptoms not recognized as being due to PMS may result in the woman being suspended from school, respite services or work, or being discouraged from being involved in recreational activities.
- When the woman is already feeling terrible due to PMS, the extra stress of behavioural management strategies being implemented may actually aggravate the symptoms.
- Stressful events such as going to the dentist or starting a new program should be avoided when the woman is premenstrual, as the woman will cope less well at that time.
- Parents who do not understand the basis of their daughter's difficult behaviour may request that she be placed in accommodation services, whereas if they view the behaviour as reflecting a medical condition that can be addressed they may be more willing to maintain their daughter at home.
- A woman who is considered behaviourally difficult may be placed with other difficult-to-manage women, a situation not only likely to aggravate her PMS symptoms, but also to deny her the quality of life she is entitled to enjoy.

For these reasons it is important to raise awareness of the range of symptoms of PMS likely to be exhibited by women with disability, particularly women who are unable to communicate effectively.

Recent data

Recent small sample research (Kyrkou, 1999) into PMS in women with an intellectual disability (data were collected from 24 women with disability – 12 with Down syndrome – plus their parents and carers) revealed that 75 per cent of the women with Down syndrome experienced pain with periods, compared with a rate of 50 per cent in women in the general population. Eight of the 12 women with Down syndrome in the sample were able to say they had pain at the time of their period. This contrasted sharply with 12 women with Autism Spectrum Disorder, only one of whom could state she had pain, yet other symptoms suggested that at least seven others were experiencing period pain sufficient to cause distress. Other symptoms considered by parents/carers of women with Down syndrome to indicate pain were facial pallor, seeming unwell, withdrawal or being unusually quiet, vomiting, cold sweats, being grumpy, crying, bending over or clutching their abdomen.

The most commonly noted symptoms of PMS and/or period pain in the sample of 12 women with Down syndrome were irritability (83 per cent), lethargy (75 per cent), crying (75 per cent), depression (67 per cent), difficulty concentrating (67 per cent), and mood swings (58 per cent). As both period pain and PMS occur premenstrually, it can be difficult to determine which symptoms are the result of which condition. One way of trying to establish whether the symptoms are more likely to be due to period pain than to PMS, is to give the woman a trial of adequate pain relief from the time the symptoms begin until the period begins. If the behaviours that are causing concern are eliminated or reduced by this treatment, it is likely that PMS is not the cause of the problems. The same approach may be taken to eliminate the symptoms due to period pain (which may coexist with PMS) in order to determine which symptoms might be due to PMS. It would be wise to consult the woman's medical practitioner, if this phase lasts more than a few days, to work out a regime of pain relief using different preparations to minimize the risk of side effects. Symptoms occurring after the period begins are more likely to be due to pain, since the rapid fall in progesterone levels which is the suspected cause of PMS has already occurred days before the period starts.

There are many treatments claimed to reduce PMS (Dalton and Holton, 1994), but none have been adequately evaluated, partly because PMS itself is hard to quantify. Relaxation of various types, avoidance of the aggravating factors listed below, or a trial of vitamin B6 or evening primrose have seemed to give most benefit. Evening primrose is not recommended for people who have epilepsy. Factors that may aggravate PMS or period pain include physical or emotional stress, disturbed or insufficient sleep, long intervals without food, excess caffeine (tea, coffee, cola, chocolate), lack of exercise, smoking (we do not know the effect of passive smoking), alcohol (especially red wine) and long-distance flights (Severino and Moline, 1989).

Concluding comment

The most important support for the woman with Down syndrome suffering premenstrually is sympathetic parents/carers who recognize what might be causing distress and seek ways to reduce it, in the meantime being sympathetic to what the woman is experiencing. Although the above issues can be seen as health issues they have many other consequences relating to education, employment and community living. They are direct issues of quality of life. Here the issues of personal perception, choice, needs and self-image are clearly present.

Study 2: Developing friendships

(Primary researchers: Verity Bottroff and Vicky Duffield)

Development of meaningful interpersonal relationships, in particular friendships, can impact greatly on a person's psychological well-being and self-worth. Friendships provide support, reassurance of personal worth, and the opportunity to express oneself and develop a sense of belonging (Heyne, 1997). One fundamental vehicle for developing friendship is through joint leisure and recreation experiences (Green and Schleien, 1991). Young people with Down syndrome, however, spend most of their time with families (Bochner and Pieterse, 1996). Amando (1993) noted that people with disabilities have fewer friends than peers who are non-disabled and there is a consequent reduction in life experience. Even when friendships are developed, the quality of the relations is different from those of their non-disabled peers (Timmons, 1993). In summary their relationships are typically limited to family members, acquaintances with disabilities and people who are paid to be with them.

The quality of life model (Romney, Brown and Fry, 1994) underscores the need to appreciate and understand personal perceptions of friendships held by adolescents with Down syndrome. Despite their developmental delay teenagers with developmental difficulties are primarily teenagers – they share a common desire for friendships with peers. There is a need to recognize their understanding of interpersonal relations in the context of their social and cognitive development, along with their communicative ability. Further their experiences in such areas as leisure and recreation would seem to be important.

This study investigated the development of friendships and the social contexts in which they may develop. Individuals' understanding of concepts associated with friendship, and difficulties associated with acquiring, developing and maintaining friends were considered. Barriers associated with friendship were highlighted along with suggestions for positive development. This included concerns experienced by parents with children who had imaginary friends. Practical implications of this study include strategies for improving the abilities of individuals with Down syndrome to develop and maintain friendships as well as providing a commentary on the role of imaginary friends.

Procedure

The study involved 20 participants with Down syndrome as well as their respective parents. Nine males and 11 females aged between 12 and 24 years took part in the study. All but two of the participants were at regular schools

(10) or at special classes or schools – one was in supported employment and another in a community support centre. Information regarding friendships was collected on an individual basis from the participants with Down syndrome using a structured interview schedule. A questionnaire was also developed from the interview schedule and sent for completion to the parents. Questions addressed the following issues: current friendship status of participants; ease in developing friendships; concepts of friendship, including imaginary friends; degree of contact with friends; and levels of engagement through various activities.

The definition of friendship used in the present study was derived from Hartup and Sancilio: that is, friendship was seen as 'reciprocity and commitment within a human relationship between individuals who see themselves as equals' (1986: 61). Using responses from both the individuals and their parents, individuals with Down syndrome were categorized into three friendship levels based on the developmental stages Selman (1980) derived from his studies on typically developing children:

Level 1 – Friendship as momentary physical interaction, e.g. you just meet the person somewhere such as at the playground or in the street.
Level 2 – Friendship as a handy playmate, e.g. someone who does what you like.
Level 3 – Friendship as mutual trust and assistance, e.g. prosocial understanding, reciprocity and sharing.

Results and discussion

In applying Selman's (1980) levels to the responses from the people with Down syndrome it was found that only 45 per cent (nine individuals) gave a response that could be analysed in terms of the levels. Inter-rater reliability for data classification was around 85 per cent. Only 25 per cent (five individuals) were classified as attaining level 3. The classification did not appear, on this small sample, to be associated with receptive language scores on the Peabody Picture Vocabulary Test-Revised (PPVT-R: Dunn and Dunn, 1981). PPVT-R scores in this group of five ranged from 4 years 1 month to 10 years 4 months with a mean of 6.3 years. The remaining 11 individuals either responded with 'Don't know' (eight individuals) or gave no verbal response at all.

Sixty per cent of the individuals (12) said it was easy to make friends, though several reasons were given for why making friends could be difficult, e.g. 'Hard – frightened', 'I'm shy,' and 'Talk to myself and because people don't like me and that'. Sixteen of the parents stated that their children had friends and 14 of these said they were within five years of the young person's own age. Most individuals were reported to have both male and female friends.

Despite this, 55 per cent of parents said their child had no special friend, a view not held by most of their children. In the nine instances of a special friend, eight of these friends had Down syndrome and one had autism. Most of the participants in the study saw their friend at school and over half also saw their friend at weekends. The activities they shared included bowling, line dancing, camps and meetings at their friends' house. Few friends were made in the community, a few at church, and a noticeable number, but below 50 per cent, were made through group activities organized particularly for individuals with Down syndrome.

Four individuals (all female) reported they had pretend or imaginary friends who were said to be with them or talked to them. Another two individuals (male) said they had imaginary friends when younger. However, eight parents noted their child with Down syndrome had imaginary friends. A female of 18 years was said to 'talk to this friend' and also replied to the friend: 'Has long and deep conversations'. Another participant (aged 14 years) even brought her imaginary friend 'to the dinner table talking to him/her'. Some individuals had multiple imaginary friends. One young woman (14 years) had four imaginary friends whom she involved in role-playing: 'she talks to them continuously and tells them her problems . . . she shouts at them'. One young man's parents said: 'He holds conversations to resolve disputes. Vents anger and frustration'.

The role of imaginary friends in the lives of those with Down syndrome needs to be considered. Is the imaginary friend primarily a feature of development, and/or a response to, or compensation for, lack of friends? With non-disabled children it is often the first born and only child, who may also be bright and creative, who develops such friends, and at preschool level, children who do not have friends tend to create imaginary ones (Manosevitz, Prentice and Wilson, 1973).

Friendship development involves a range of concepts and skills beyond knowing what makes a friend, such as how to make friends and how to resolve conflicts. There is probably a need to teach specific skills associated with making and maintaining friendships. There is a need to develop concepts of friendship through practical example and this is most likely to occur if at least some non-disabled peers are involved. There is also the need to practise 'making friends', which in the case of non-disabled children is able to take place from a very young age. These suggestions raise issues of school inclusion and, at a later age, normal employment environments, since with more non-disabled peers around both opportunity and example may occur.

It is one thing to have specific knowledge about friendship, another to develop a friendship network. Brown, Bayer and Brown (1992) noted that some adults with disabilities, including those with Down syndrome, developed friendships spontaneously when in the community, after experiencing opportunities to exercise choices and select activities which they personally identified. Of course, this cannot be done easily unless there is a wide range of environmental opportunity.

In the present study around 50 per cent of friendships were made at school. The other half appeared to have been made in the context of groups for people with Down syndrome, with only a few being made in the neighbourhood. It is perhaps obvious that people are more likely to make friends in the places were they spend large amounts of their time. Thus, until people with Down syndrome have a wider range of normal peer group environments in which to meet, they are likely to make friends only with other people with Down syndrome. This would appear appropriate, but a leavening of friends from other groups is likely to encourage greater understanding and development of friendships and to increase an individual's levels of performance and opportunities for choice, thus increasing self-image and motivation.

Easy and regular access to community settings would provide the opportunity for individuals with Down syndrome to feel comfortable in such environments, which to some extent is associated with a degree of familiarity. Parents noted that their child was 'reluctant to make friends', 'doesn't look for friendship activities' or 'prefers to be on his own'. This reluctance, along with the difficulties that some parents had in 'organizing contact outside school' or involving their child in events organized for those with Down syndrome, highlights the challenges involved in providing regular and normal peer venues. Despite the difficulties described by some parents, about one third of the sample had frequent contact with friends (i.e. every night or once or twice a week).

Many children with Down syndrome appear to develop imaginary friends and it seems likely that some of this may be attributed to the developmental process, and some to the lack of contact or opportunity for friends. It is probable that such behaviour is likely to reduce when an array of stable friendships can develop. It is apparent that some parents are concerned or embarrassed at the development of such friendships but they do represent compensation and provide opportunity for play and for the practice of language. As described later in this chapter the development of imagination and mental imagery represents important aspects of learning, particularly in the social and cognitive spheres, and is to be accepted rather than stifled.

Concluding comment

In this study the issues of quality of life are seen as critical concepts against which we need to assess studies of friendship development and underline why that development is so critical to long-term well-being. For example, it has relevance to issues surrounding personal longevity since individuals surrounded and supported by friends are more likely to survive and have quality experiences than are individuals who, having lost parents in later life, are very much isolated.

Study 3: Challenges to employment: perceptions and barriers as seen by people with Down syndrome and their parents

(Primary researchers: John Grantley, Roy Brown and Judy Thornley)

This research is based on a quality of life and well-being model (see Brown et al., 1992 and Goode, 1994) and is concerned with the expressed choices and preferences of people with Down syndrome regarding their post-school life experience. It is particularly concerned with the perceptions of young people with Down syndrome and their parents.

Procedure

Fourteen young people with Down syndrome, nine females and five males, aged between 18 and 30 years, were interviewed before they obtained employment. Parents were also sent a questionnaire, and similar questions were asked in both instances. Monitoring continues as individuals progress towards open employment. This paper explores issues such as the individuals' reasons for wanting employment and where they would like to be employed. The type of work experience provided at school, perceived barriers to employment and the perceived need for further training were also explored.

Results and discussion

In considering the responses from the two groups involved in the study some differences were apparent. People with Down syndrome emphasized their reasons for wanting work. They were interested in having the opportunity to perform specific tasks or valued roles in employment and, to a lesser extent, establishing relationships and improving their personal well-being. Their parents or carers tended to emphasize the need for personal development, in terms of independence, self-esteem and personal well-being, e.g. 'To maintain a level of self-esteem and independence'.

Parents were more concerned about the person and their level of satisfaction than about the type or status of the employment. The people with Down syndrome, on the other hand, were more concerned with the type of work they would like to perform, that is, their thinking was more direct and concrete. Some examples of the responses made to questions about future employment were: 'Because I'll be able to be a nurse'; 'I will be helping – make food, washing dishes'.

One of the challenges set by the quality of life model is to recognize that young people with Down syndrome will make specific choices. These need to be understood and accepted while helping them to understand some of the more complex reasons for work and that employment is only likely if they get experience of real work. Parents tended to select the more traditional types of jobs considered suitable for people with intellectual disabilities, whereas those with Down syndrome suggested a wider range of employment possibilities. The jobs nominated by parents could be fitted into 10 categories, whereas 17 categories were required to contain the choices of the individuals with Down syndrome. There was more variation in job choice amongst people with Down syndrome than their parents and the additional preferences nominated by some people with Down syndrome included jobs in which people with Down syndrome are actually employed (e.g. dancer, waiter, factory worker, shop assistant). This suggests that more attention might be given to the individual's own choices.

Most parents, in line with modern approaches, hoped for open employment with or without support, though about a third thought that a sheltered workshop was the most likely option. Given data on the individuals' skill levels this would probably be an underestimate of what individuals could do. Yet work experience arranged by the individuals' schools was restricted to school-based or sheltered employment for around 50 per cent of the group. Educational authorities need to find ways to broaden experiences in employment while the child is still enrolled in school.

For these broader experiences to be successful, further training would be required, although this could possibly be accomplished in the context of the work experience. When considering necessary skills other than those directly related to the work tasks, people with Down syndrome and their parents or carers emphasized similar areas including social skills, self-help skills, grooming, independent living skills, academic skills and budget training. People with Down syndrome also emphasized the need to develop friendship skills and social skills. Parents put a little more emphasis on marriage preparation, an issue that should be considered for part of the educational curriculum. The data also point to the fact that parents should be consulted and involved actively in the transition period from school to work. Frequently, skills are not specific work skills, but those skills which are related to a person's quality of life, including their self-esteem and personal well-being. But we know effective quality of life is based on an holistic or integrated approach to learning and performance, and should be taught in a fashion that recognizes this.

Although people with Down syndrome and their parents were able to clearly state their perceived training requirements, only 56 per cent of the parents and 28 per cent of the people with Down syndrome indicated that they knew where to access vocational training. Riches states emphatically that there is a 'lack of information on just what services are available post-school, as well as an inadequate number of appropriate high quality adult services' (1996: 430). Where appropriate vocational training is currently available, it needs to be documented, publicized in plain English and disseminated through schools and disability service agencies, to all relevant consumers and their families.

Concluding comment

This report has shown that if people with Down syndrome and their parents are asked their opinions about current and future employment expectations and aspirations, they are able to give positive and optimistic responses that are wide ranging and challenging. It is suggested that the preferences of people with Down syndrome, as well as those of their parents, are given high priority when considering employment opportunities, particularly in the selection of work experience and the location of those work experience placements. When seeking employment opportunities for people with Down syndrome, their preferences and choices should be given the most serious consideration and perhaps higher priority than those of their parents and teachers. People do best when given control of choices, though experience may modify these choices. This applies to persons with Down syndrome, as well as their parents and teachers. To satisfy vocational preferences of the people with Down syndrome and their parents, it is suggested that more consumer-influenced vocational programs be developed (Agran, Test and Martin, 1994).

Finally, the currently available vocational training programs should be publicized widely to ensure all consumers are well informed. People with Down syndrome have shown that they are able to articulate their aspirations, preferences and needs for their working lives. If they are provided with the relevant information regarding available vocational opportunities and training programs then they will be able to make more informed and effective choices, giving them more control over their future employment opportunities. These are significant characteristics that contribute to an improved quality of life for people with Down syndrome, not only during their later school years but also when they are adults in the workforce who will eventually face retirement without, in most instances, the availability of parents.

Study 4: Mental imagery in Down syndrome – a new door to development?

(Primary researchers: Roy Brown and Eddie Bullitis)

There has been little work carried out that incorporates both mental imagery and disability (see Courbois, 1996), and none on Down syndrome which is known to the authors (but see our previous report: Brown and Bullitis, 1998). Yet many interventions, programmes and counselling approaches seem to imply that mental imagery processes are present in all individuals (Groden et al., 1991). We believe that mental imagery is likely to be at least useful, if not essential, for a variety of educational, social and other developmental changes. Mental imagery may be valuable in learning and performing activities of daily living, creative activities such as music and arts, education and problem solving, and in the use of imagination in making choices. But it is not even known whether some or all persons with developmental disabilities experience mental imagery.

Procedure

The present study was exploratory and investigated the process of imagery in people with developmental disabilities, but this paper particularly comments on people with Down syndrome. The questions for the study were: 'Does everybody have mental imagery?'; 'Can imagery be manipulated?'; and 'What are its possible roles in individuals' development?'

The participants were 16 adult individuals with intellectual disabilities (five with Down syndrome) and 10 undergraduate students. Participants were seen individually and shown nine pictures for brief periods of time (10 seconds each). The pictures showed such scenes as a man blowing out birthday candles. After each presentation the participant was asked to reply to a series of questions, such as: 'What did you see?'; 'Can you imagine the person talking?'; 'Can you talk to him/her?'; 'Can you make him/her climb a ladder?'; 'What does this feel like?' Participants were videotaped throughout the session so that motor, visual and verbal behaviours could be recorded. Prior to this procedure each individual's understanding was checked for words such as *chair*, *box*, *car*, *mind*, and *think* that were used in the questioning.

Results and discussion

The responses from each person were examined and individuals compared. Although we cannot assume that imagery does or does not take place, some individuals appeared to report clear imagery, and others were unable to make responses in relation to imagining situations. Those who made responses frequently showed motor and eye movements consistent with the imagery. However, in this group there was considerable variation amongst individuals, particularly those with Down syndrome, with several verbalizing graphic imagery, some with considerable excitement and elaboration. Such individuals were often able to enter the imaginative scene playing a variety of roles and experiencing types of imagery beyond the visual (i.e. auditory and tactile). It seems possible that such abilities are a considerable aid to learning. If this behaviour is to be utilized it will be important to examine further the process itself, the behaviours of the guide or instructor who implements the process, and the characteristics of the process in the individual who receives instruction.

A few responses from one of the pictures presented to the participants illustrate some of these points. The picture involved a woman in overalls standing by a ladder with a cup in her hand. After removal of the picture, and following some preliminary questions, participants were asked whether they could put themselves in the picture and climb the ladder. One response was:

No, I can't.
Why not?
Because I can't, because I'm scared of heights.

Another person said she couldn't climb the ladder because 'I might fall'. A participant in responding to another picture said she could not stand by a fire and warm her hands 'because it is dangerous'.

Such responses not only suggest strong mental imagery, but raise issues about how individuals make social responses and how environmental experiences represent themselves in imagery, thus possibly inhibiting or exciting responses. In other scenarios some individuals denied imagery and could make no responses to 'imagery provoking' questions while in another instance an individual indicated that visual imagery was possible when he was young but he no longer experienced such imagery. Here questions are raised about the effects of experience and deprivation. (How does experience promote imagery and what role does it play in development?) This highlights issues of concern regarding institutionalization, environmental deprivation, restricting risk-taking opportunities, etc. It seems reasonable to hypothesize that such situations might inhibit or reduce imagery processes or increase anxiety-making images. Stimulation, experience and increasing control over the environment might be expected to both enhance imagery and also promote imagery as an important control agent in behaviour.

The apparent tendency for richer imagery amongst persons with Down syndrome, compared with other people with intellectual disabilities, may reflect a greater capacity for fantasy, which in turn may be related to environmental stimulation, a variety of life experiences, and rich and supportive family and social networks. Some individuals with Down syndrome sometimes displayed vivid mental imagery. It was noted that such individuals had often been involved in drama, where imagery techniques are utilized in rehearsal. Does this have implications for learning strategies, with possible relevance to various life domains (e.g. in teaching socially appropriate behaviour)? Again, the opposite conditions might be expected to be associated with reduced imagery - exclusion processes including, for example, institutionalization and nonintegrated classes - the data showed the effects of environmental experience. It was also apparent that some individuals showed changes in the type of statements about mental imagery as the research proceeded. This could have been related to an increase in the individual's awareness or familiarity with the situation. Yet an examination of responses suggests some were surprised, as they found it possible to imagine specific scenes or events. Examples were given of individuals sensing sound, smell and taste, though these were less common than visual responses.

It seems possible that professionals make assumptions about people's conscious awareness and also the potential role it may play in learning and development. In the field of disabilities, at least, understanding of awareness and mental imagery seems to be in its infancy. In this context it is believed that imagery should not be forced where it induces anxiety, but it would seem to have possible positive effects in enhancing social learning and formal education. However, the amount of variation amongst individuals suggests its use must be explored on an individual basis. Therefore, it is necessary to consider how techniques might be developed to improve imagery processes amongst those with intellectual disabilities and help people, such as some of those with Down syndrome, who have good mental imagery processes, to use them more effectively.

It is recognized that the processes described are difficult to measure, which makes us cautious in coming to conclusions. Indeed the material raised here should be treated as ideas for further exploration. The authors accept that what individuals say about themselves and their imagery is a reasonably reliable reflection of their perceptions. They are accounts of what individuals believe they are visualizing or imaging. The content of the ideas suggests the accounts are both spontaneous and, at times, elaborate. Some individuals experienced major challenges. For example, there were individuals who said, 'I did get a picture but now it's gone, I keep on trying but I can't get it'. Other individuals recognized that they previously possessed the skill of mental imagery, but that skill was now lost. Is such a loss due to ageing processes, or loss of stimulation? Answers to such questions may have implications for lifestyle and rehabilitation. The relevance of these observations needs to be explored further, particularly in relation to development and learning. If it is agreed that the process of mental imagery is critical, then it is crucial to:

- explore the topic further;
- consider the use of imagery on an individual basis (observe and promote);
- consider developing various educational and training techniques to improve people's imagery.

Concluding comment

In this study the questions concerning mental imagery arose directly from quality of life studies. The sensitization provided from such a conceptualiza- tion led to an accent on individual variation and how individuals went about improving their well-being. There is an aspect to quality of life that helps us concentrate on detail and draws attention to individuals rather than groups, and encourages us to pose questions about how and why individuals respond differently. The concepts posed at the beginning of the chapter can be directed to the issue of mental imagery and how the presence or absence of such a process may help or hinder the individual's quality of life. Further, if mental imagery is absent or ill developed, it is necessary to discover how it can be developed and improved. These are research questions which have yet to be clearly answered. However, the authors suggest the issues are important to learning and development and as such are important considera- tions for parents and professionals.

Concluding remarks

In the above studies the authors have used a model or blueprint referred to as quality of life. It is one of a number of models, but it has been used here to encourage the authors to look at challenges in understanding the lives of those with Down syndrome in different ways and to pose questions to our audience. It is believed that society needs to look at individuals with Down syndrome in a rather more integrated fashion and to pull together specific studies in such a way that systems and practices can be developed in order for a lifespan and holistic approach to the challenges to be developed at a personal level.

Friendships in childhood and adolescence enable individuals to function more effectively as adults; self-image rises when individuals' premenstrual stress is taken into account and remedies are developed; increased choices over employment and the encouragement of employment make individuals more stable and independent; and the encouragement of mental imagery may lead to better developed cognitive and emotional processes. The current studies are necessarily only examples of possible undertakings that use a quality of life framework, each of which has been carried out with the help of people with Down syndrome and their parents. It is to be hoped that studies from such a perspective will enable parents of children with Down syndrome to see their children as people of value and potential who are likely to grow into adults who recognize themselves as contributors to society. The interesting sideline to this is that the quality of life perspective enables the messages involved to be seen as applicable to all children, and thus the label of disability is replaced by one of individual variation.

Acknowlegements

We acknowledge our gratitude to the individuals who took part in these studies and the support of the Down Syndrome Association of South Australia Inc. and Interwork Limited, Adelaide.

References

Agran M, Test D, Martin J (1994) Employment preparation of students with severe disabilities. In Cipano E, Spooner F (Eds) Curricular and Instructional Approaches for Persons with Severe Disabilities. Massachusetts: Allyn and Bacon.

Amando AN (1993) Friendships and Community Connections Between People With and Without Developmental Disabilities. Sydney: Paul H. Brookes.

Bochner S, Pieterse M (1996) Teenagers with Down syndrome in a time of changing policies and practices: progress of students who were born between 1971 and 1978. International Journal of Disabilities, Development and Education 43: 75-95.

Brown RI (1997) Quality of Life for People With Disabilities. Cheltenham: Stanley Thornes.

Brown RI, Bayer MB, Brown PM (1992) Empowerment and Developmental Handicaps: Choices and Quality of Life. Toronto, Ontario: Captus Press.

Brown RI, Bullitis E (1998) Images of consciousness: some preliminary notes on mental imagery. In Virji-Babul N, Kisly D (Eds) Down Syndrome in the 21st Century. Vancouver: Down Syndrome Research Foundation and Resource Centre. pp 76-82.

Courbois Y (1996) Evidence for visual imagery defects in persons with mental retardation. American Journal on Mental Retardation 101: 130-48.

Cummins RA (1997) Assessing quality of life. In RI Brown (Ed) Quality of Life for People with Disabilities: Models, Research and Practice. Cheltenham: Stanley Thornes. pp 116-50.

Dalton K, Holton D (1994) PMS: The Essential Guide to Treatment Options. London: Thorsons.

Dunn LM, Dunn LM (1981) Peabody Picture Vocabulary test - Revised. Circle Pines, MN: American Guidance Services.

Frank RT (1931) The hormonal causes of premenstrual tension. Archives of Neurology and Psychiatry 26: 1053-7.

Goode DA (1994) Quality of Life for Persons with Disabilities: International Perspectives and Issues. Cambridge, MA: Brookline.

Green FP, Schleien SJ (1991) Understanding friendship and recreation: a theoretical sampling. Therapeutic Recreation Journal 25(4): 29-40.

Groden J, Cautela JR, LeVasseur P, Groden G, Bausman M (1991) Imagery Procedures for People with Special Needs: Breaking the Barriers II, Video Guide. Illinois: Research Press.

Hartup WW, Sancilio MF (1986) Children's friendships. In Scholar E, Mesibov GB (Eds) Social Behaviour and Autism. New York: Plenum Press.

Heyne LA (1997) Friendship. In Schleien SJ, Ray MT, FP Green (Eds) Community Recreation and People with Disabilities. Sydney: Paul H. Brookes.

IASSID (2000) Quality of Life - Its Conceptualization, Measurement and Application: A Consensus Document - Report to the International Association for the Scientific Study of Intellectual Disability. Seattle: IASSID.

Kyrkou MR (1999) Description of PMS symptoms in women with disability. Unpublished dissertation for Master of Disability Studies, Flinders University, Adelaide, Australia.

Manosevitz M, Prentice NM, Wilson F (1973) Individual and family correlates of imaginary companions in preschool children. Developmental Psychology 8: 72-9.

Mortola JF (1995) In Carr PL, Freund KM, Somani S (Eds) The Medical Care of Women. Philadelphia: W.B. Saunders. pp 191-200.

Renwick R, Brown I (1996) The Centre for Health Promotion's conceptual approach to quality of life. In Renwick R, Brown I, Nagler M (Eds) Quality of Life in Health Promotion and Rehabilitation: Conceptual Approaches, Issues and Applications. Thousand Oaks, CA: Sage Publications. pp 75-86.

Riches V (1996) Transition from school to community. In Stratford B, Gunn P (Eds) New Approaches to Down Syndrome. London: Cassell. pp 424-35.

Romney DM, Brown RI, Fry PS (1994) Improving the quality of life: prescriptions for change. In Romney DR, Brown RI, Fry PS (Eds) Improving the Quality of Life; Recommendations for People With and Without Disabilities. Dordrecht, Netherlands: Kluwer.

Selman RL (1980) The Growth of Interpersonal Understanding: Development and Clinical Analyses. New York: Academic Press.

Severino SK, Moline ML (1989) Premenstrual Syndrome: A Clinician's Guide. New York: The Guilford Press.

Timmons V (1993) Quality of life of teenagers with special needs. Unpublished doctoral dissertation, University of Calgary, Canada.

CHAPTER 11
From autonomy to work placement

ANNA CONTARDI

The Associazione Italiana Persone Down (the Italian Association for Down Syndrome People: AIPD) is an association for people with Down syndrome and their families which is a reference point in Italy for parents and for all who are involved in this field. Its aim is to provide information to parents and others about Down syndrome and to promote initiatives to improve the situation of people with Down syndrome. In recent years it has increasingly devoted attention to the needs of adults with Down syndrome (Contardi and Vicari, 1994). As is now well known, the average life expectancy of people with Down syndrome has increased and it is calculated that of the 49 000 individuals with Down syndrome in Italy, 30 000 are over the age of 18 (Mastroiacovo et al., 1997). One consequence of this awareness has been that the association has changed its name from Associazione Bambini Down (the Down Children's Association) to Associazione Italiana Persone Down (the Italian Association for Down Syndrome People). In addition, the association has begun projects and is providing services that focus on adults.

One project begun by the AIPD is an educational course that has the aim of increasing social autonomy in people with Down syndrome (Contardi, 1992). Social autonomy (for example, the ability to handle money, find one's way, use public transport and public services) was chosen as a focus as these skills are seen to be important if individuals with Down syndrome are to be included in the normal social context, which, for adults, includes the workplace (Hobart, 1996). The first course was organized with the Rome branch of the AIPD in 1989 and was designed for adolescents and adults ranging in age from 15 to 20. Since 1989 the course has been repeated every year with increasing numbers and has been adopted in many other cities. Since the course was first brought into being over 200 teenagers with Down syndrome have taken part in courses in Rome and in other Italian cities.

The educational course for the acquisition of social autonomy takes the form of a series of weekly meetings (about three hours each) in the teenager's free time. Each adolescent meets with a group made up of eight to nine people with Down syndrome and three to four social workers. After a joint session the group divides up into subgroups of two to three people with Down syndrome, plus a social worker and a volunteer worker.

The educational objectives proposed by the programme can be grouped into five areas:

- communication;
- orientation;
- road behaviour;
- using money;
- shopping and more generally making use of services.

Success in these areas is sought by concentrating on specific activities such as going bowling, going out for a pizza, shopping, paying bills at the post office and so on, where the young people 'learn by doing' in a context that is appropriate for their age. The educators devote a great deal of attention to the motivation of the teenagers, the authenticity of the situations that are proposed and the individualization of objectives and educational strategies.

With varying degrees of success, all the youngsters who have participated have made progress. All of them are now able to cross roads by themselves, use a public telephone, ask for information in order to resolve their difficulties and, within certain limits, all know how to go shopping for minor items. Furthermore, there are aspects of personality in each of them, such as self-confidence, self-esteem, and the capacity to establish relations with others, where noticeable improvement in knowledge and structural development in their own identities can be noted (aspects of personal autonomy). All who have participated in the program left the program seeing themselves as teenagers capable of doing a wide variety of things, albeit with certain limitations (Contardi, 1998).

Description of an alliance with a company aimed at increasing the employment of young people with Down syndrome

In Italy it is compulsory for companies with more than 35 workers to employ individuals with a disability. Although the law exists, many companies do what they can to avoid employing a person with an intellectual disability, whether out of concern for problems of inclusion or because they believe that such a person will not be productive. To a large extent this is due to prejudice, but also to the fact that the law has not provided any incentives for companies to employ individuals with a disability; nor does there exist a specifically aimed employment scheme to ensure that the worker chosen for the post has the training necessary for that job (Lepri, Montobbio and Papone, 1999). The law has recently been modified to include these points but it is not yet operative.

In 1992 the AIPD published the results of a survey of 34 people with Down syndrome in the workplace (Sampaolo and Danesi, 1993). The authors identified three key elements that were necessary for a successful work placement – good personal/social autonomy in the individual worker; a good match between the demands of the job and the worker's skills; and on-the-job training. These three elements provided the basis for the major aspects of the work placement program developed by the AIPD. First, the program aimed to develop a good level of personal/social autonomy in each worker, and then concentrated on choosing the appropriate job, followed by in-service training. This has required that the AIPD contacts companies directly, in order to work with them to find an inclusion procedure that satisfies both sides.

With these aims in mind AIPD has been working since 1993 with Food Italia, a company that runs five McDonald's restaurants in Rome. Food Italia is a company that is obliged by law to employ workers with disabilities, but it has often experienced difficulty at the inclusion phase with the people who were sent by the Employment Office of the Province, an office which deals with unemployed groups.

The first step in successfully matching a job and a worker is an evaluation of the job and then an evaluation of the candidate(s) for that job (Montobbio, 1993). An analysis of the tasks required of a worker in a McDonald's restaurant showed that the workplace includes a variety of tasks that range from the preparation of food, to cleaning, to serving the members of the public. A profile of the personal characteristics an individual would need to be successful in the workplace was also drawn up, keeping the tasks identified above in mind. These included:

- personal cleanliness (particularly important when there is contact with food and with the general public);
- the ability to reach the workplace independently because the work involves different shifts;
- the capacity to ask for help in case of difficulty;
- the capacity to carry out simple instructions.

The ability to read and write was considered useful, but not essential for successful functioning in this workplace. It is apparent that almost all these characteristics require a degree of personal or social autonomy.

The company and those working with the young people with Down syndrome next considered the organization of the job. It was decided together that the contract should be a part-time training contract (20 hours per week). The training contract is widely used in Italy for the employment of young people as it offers a series of tax advantages for the company. It lasts for 2 years, after which time it can be terminated or transformed into a permanent contract. This kind of contract was already used by the company for other workers, as indeed was the part-time contract. The latter is ideal for many people with Down syndrome as it eliminates the problem of their becoming excessively tired. Work in a fast-food restaurant is considerably more tiring than in many other work situations. The only concession made was to fix the daily working hours and the day off for the worker with Down syndrome. Other workers change shift on a regular basis. This measure was taken to ensure that the worker with Down syndrome was as independent as possible as far as getting public transport to work was concerned. Workers with Down syndrome earn the same salary as other workers doing similar jobs.

Almost immediately this cooperative venture had begun, the company felt the need for someone to deal specifically with the training of workers with special needs and so the position of 'job coach' was created. The characteristics considered necessary for this role were a good knowledge of the work and of the training schemes, a basic knowledge of psychology, and the ability to listen and to observe. The choice of person for this job was made jointly by Food Italia's Head of Personnel and the staff member of the AIPD who was monitoring the project. A young manager was chosen who was subsequently given a short course at the AIPD and who continues to refer to the AIPD staff member for supervision and help in specific areas (Lodico, 1999).

As part of the agreement with the company, AIPD undertook to select potential candidates in order to have a pool of possible workers on which to draw every time a post became vacant. Given the requirements mentioned above it was felt to be important that the candidates should have taken part in the AIPD's Acquisition of Autonomy course. Almost all the young people selected for work had attended such a course, which proved extremely useful both because they had acquired specific abilities and because they had developed an ability to relate well with colleagues and managers.

When a job vacancy arises the company notifies the AIPD worker(s), who in turn identify possible candidates. The company holds a series of job interviews, including interviewing candidates without a disability. In the case of a young person with Down syndrome, the job coach and the representative of the AIPD are also present. If the young person is selected for the position, the necessary bureaucratic procedures are completed and the individual is employed on a training contract.

In the initial period the job coach is often present to supervise the training procedure, to help the individual with Down syndrome to carry out the tasks he or she has been assigned, and to help in his or her role as a worker. The training period provides the worker with Down syndrome with the possibility of gradually learning all the tasks that the job involves, although the order in which the tasks are taught may vary from the usual sequence and the time necessary for learning may be longer than suggested by the training manual. After the initial period (varying with each individual case) the job coach steps back, spending only one day a week in the same McDonald's as the young person to encourage greater autonomy, while at the same time remaining a point of reference.

Initially the simplest tasks, such as cleaning, serving at the drinks station and stacking the shelves, are taught. These have been selected in order to increase self-confidence and, with this, the desire to work. The next stage is the learning of more complex tasks, from the various kitchen tasks to working at the cash desk, although the time scale and the methods used vary from case to case according to the individual and the needs of the company. The young people with Down syndrome use all the machinery, including high temperature fryers.

From the first day the young person is expected to consider the job seriously, to arrive punctually, to show respect for the rules and towards his or her colleagues, to take orders from superiors, to be polite to the public and generally to carry out the different tasks efficiently. That is to say, they are expected to perform the job in the same way as other workers.

Outcomes of the employment project

Between 1994 and 1998 eight workers with Down syndrome were given jobs in a McDonald's restaurant. All continue to be employed. Table 11.1 provides a description of the educational, training and work experience of the young people with Down syndrome, prior to their employment.

All eight of the young people had a good level of autonomy and they quickly learnt how to reach work on their own, taking one or two forms of public transport. As far as learning the different tasks is concerned there have been no particular problems, although not all have yet learned to use the till. The job coach has placed most emphasis on helping the workers with Down syndrome to comprehend the particular requests made of them and to understand why the various actions required of them are necessary. AIPD was involved primarily in the early phases to help colleagues in the restaurant to understand that the worker with Down syndrome was first and foremost a worker like themselves and to understand any specific difficulties that they might have.

Table 11.1 The educational, training and work experience of the eight young people with Down syndrome who were employed in a McDonald's restaurant

Gender and age	Year of placement	School and training experience	Previous work experience
Female 23 yrs	1993	Middle school[a]	None
Male 24 yrs	1995	Secondary school[b], post-school agricultural course, related practical experience	None
Male 25 yrs	1995	Middle school, hotel and catering course	None
Female 31 yrs	1996	Middle school, practical experience	None
Male 23 yrs	1997	Middle school, hotel and catering course, practical experience	Experience of factory work which ended when the factory closed down
Female 23 yrs	1998	Hotel and catering school, computer training course	None
Male 23 yrs	1998	Middle school, office training course, day centre	None
Female 26 yrs	1998	Middle school, office training course, day centre	None

[a]Middle school – generally attended by children between the ages of 11 and 13 years.
[b]Secondary school – generally attended by children between the ages of 14 and 18 years.

The company has recently carried out an evaluation of productivity and has found that the productivity of these workers is between 70 and 80 per cent of that of other workers. This is a very important result and it suggests the methodology chosen for the inclusion procedure is an effective one. It also refutes the idea that employment for a person with special needs is a form of social assistance.

There are several aspects of the McDonald's organization that helped contribute to the success of the venture. The training contract implies a certain amount of in-service training and McDonald's has developed a manual and a well-structured training scheme for all its workers. Each work station, such as 'Salads', 'Drinks' etc., has a specific work procedure which everyone follows in every McDonald's restaurant. All of these supports can also usefully be used with people with Down syndrome. Other characteristics of the organization that helped contribute to the successful integration of the individuals with Down syndrome include the fact that there is a clear hierarchical order, where the roles of manager, director etc. are very clear, giving easily identifiable points of reference; and the policy requiring workers to wear a uniform helped the young people with Down syndrome to feel that they belonged to the company and to identify with the role of worker.

It is clear from the behaviour of the young people involved in this scheme that their new status as worker has had a positive effect on their self-confidence. The fact that they feel grown up and are recognized as such, and that they are bringing home a salary has meant that their behaviour both at home and with their friends is more adult and more responsible. This is still more evident in the cases where the families have allowed them to be responsible for the money they have earned, although this is always under supervision. One young person has opened a bank account and uses a bancomat/ cashpoint card; another has bought a mobile telephone, which he uses competently and appropriately. Most have started to do new things, such as going to a beautician's or organizing evenings with friends.

Relationships with colleagues are generally good, and in some cases excellent. In a recent report a company manager has written:

> My impression is that the arrival of these new employees has widened the general consciousness, brought more understanding and harmony, and an appreciation of other colleagues that was difficult to find before . . . many of their colleagues have become friends. They go out together for a pizza or to celebrate someone's birthday or just to chat about boyfriends, girlfriends, clothes or football.

This is the story of one worker with Down syndrome:

> My first day of work was on Monday at 4 o'clock. I saw the restaurant and the manager and I tried on the uniform and met my colleagues. I was nervous. On Monday, Thursday, Friday and Sunday I work from 3 o'clock until 7 o'clock. On Wednesday I work from 10 to 2 (because in the afternoon I go swimming), and Tuesday and Saturday are my free days. Every day I clock in when I arrive and I clock out when I finish work, before I go away.
>
> With my colleagues everything's fine. They work different shifts, the night shift too. I do my job by myself and they help me when I need it. I prepare all the kinds of burgers, and I do the training till – the manager helps me and explains how the till works. I prepare the drinks, the chips, the ice-creams, the apple pies and I make the milk shakes and the sundaes, which is a kind of ice-cream, and I do the cones with cream. When I work in the morning I do the salad bar, where the salads are sold, I take the orders, I put them on the plates, I take the money at the till.

Another says:

> My salary is paid into the bank so when I need money I use bancomat. I buy myself things – smart clothes, shoes with high heels, jackets and shirts, and I go to the theatre and to the cinema or have a pizza with my friends. Since I've been working my life has got better – I've changed as a person, I've grown up, become an adult. I've become a woman.

Conclusion

Though not all people with Down syndrome may be able to work, for a great many of them employment is a possible objective. The company structure of McDonald's has been a positive element in the success of the initiative described in this chapter. It seems clear that it is not the type of work itself, but rather the organization of the work that is the reason for this success and that this organization can be applied to other work environments. Another element that would seem to be indispensable for success is an appropriate level of personal and social autonomy in the young person with Down syndrome. Achieving this autonomy involves all who are responsible for their upbringing: the family, the school, and those who assist in organizing their free-time activities.

The AIPD's work placement scheme described here is, without doubt, an anomalous service in that it is promoted by a private body, but the functions it has carried out in this trial are typical of any service engaged in work placement for individuals with an intellectual disability. The experience described here can provide a guideline for developing specifically chosen job placements as well as a model for cooperation between social services or other placement organizations and a company willing to employ workers with an intellectual disability. Finally, it must be stated that in recent years we have tried to promote similar schemes with other companies, not always with the same good results. We are determined, however, to continue to push for increased employment opportunities for individuals with Down syndrome and to develop the support systems that will enhance the likelihood of their success.

References

Contardi A (1992) Libertà Possibile. Roma: La Nuova Italia Scientifica ed.

Contardi A (1998) The educational course in the acquisition of the autonomy of Associazione Italiana Persone Down. Down Syndrome Research and Practice 16: 93-8.

Contardi A, Vicari S (1994) Le Persone Down, Aspetti Neuropsicologici, Educativi e Sociali. Milano: Franco Angeli ed.

Hobart Zambon A (1996) La Persona con Sindrome di Down: Un'introduzione per la sua famiglia. Roma: Il Pensiero Scientifico ed.

Lepri C, Montobbio E, Papone G (1999) Lavori in Corso. Tirrenia: Del Cerro ed.

Lodico G (1999) Finalmente un vero lavoro. Appunti sulle politiche sociali 121(2): 6-9.

Mastroiacovo P et al. (1997) Epidemiologia e qualita di vita: alcuni dati in Italia. In la persona Down verso il 2000: un nuovo soggetto sociale. Roma: Associazione Italiana Persone Down. pp xix-xxxi.

Montobbio E (1993) Lavoro e Fasce Deboli. Milano: Franco Angeli ed.

Sampaolo E, Danesi P (1993) Un Posto per Tutti. Pisa: Del Cerro ed.

SECTION 6
FAMILIES

Introduction

As the chapter by Jobling and Cuskelly in the section on adult life makes clear, parents of individuals with Down syndrome often have responsibilities for their child well beyond the age when most offspring have established independent lives for themselves. This is not unique to parents of a child with Down syndrome, but is a common experience for parents of a child with a disability. Services that support independent living are less well developed than are educational services, at least in Australia, and this means that parents' lives are more likely to differ from that of their age peers at this time of their life than at earlier stages. This may have some negative effects on parents, but, as Susanne Muirhead's chapter makes clear, it is unwarranted to assume all parents find this entirely burdensome.

Muirhead's chapter provides a refreshing approach to the experience of having a child with Down syndrome. In her introductory section she reveals details of her own life which she sees as having been important in deciding the direction her research would take. She suggests that we too readily accept that the difference in parenting patterns experienced by parents of adults with a disability is an altogether negative experience. She presents evidence that for some parents, at least, there is not the case. The parents who participated in her study made it clear that their present view did not reflect their initial response to having a child with Down syndrome - they reported that they came to their current accommodation as a gradual process. Parents saw their child with Down syndrome as a person who had helped them learn - about themselves, the world, other ways of seeing. Finally, parents expressed joy in the caring relationship they experienced with their child.

The following paper by Monica Cuskelly, Anne Jobling, David Chant, Anna Bower, and Alan Hayes discusses several aspects of family life - maternal experiences and concerns, parents' experience of stress and the relationship between the individual with Down syndrome and his or her siblings. Different methods were used to collect the information presented here, and informants also differed: in one study only mothers were included; in another both parents' views were collected; and in the study on sibling relationships the views of mothers, fathers and children were sought. There were also commonalities across the studies - each tried to broaden the information about family life, either through methods of data collection or the number of informants, and each allowed space for positive outcomes to emerge. For many years, research on family life was restricted to collecting the views of mothers. They are important but the perspectives of other family members need to be understood equally well if a clear and complete view of family life is to be gained. Where appropriate, the family member with Down syndrome should also be asked to contribute her or his opinions. There is little research available on family life where the person with Down syndrome has been invited to contribute. However, as Jan Gothard's earlier chapter illustrates, this may be changing.

CHAPTER 12
An appreciative inquiry about adults with Down syndrome

SUSANNE MUIRHEAD

Introduction

Down syndrome is one of the most frequently occurring chromosomal anomalies found in humans and has become one of the most controversial, researched and discussed genetic variations of human kind. Over the past 100 years, since the label 'Down syndrome' came into existence, the working language used to describe Down syndrome provides enlightening insight on how Down syndrome has come to be generally understood: Mongoloid idiocy; imperfection in DNA; foetal abnormality; severe affliction; chromosomic abnormality; disorder; severe, disabling, genetic disease (see, for example, McDonough, 1990; Stratford, 1991; Williams, 1995). Stratford (1991) states that even though by the turn of the century the condition was being referred to as Down's syndrome, the term Mongol persisted in the literature until well into the 1970s, and to this day has not entirely disappeared from the language. People with Down syndrome have been represented with labels such as: a drain on resources, deficient, Mongoloid idiots, impaired, unproductive, inadequate, mentally retarded, mentally handicapped, disabled, slow, a lifelong burden (see, for example, Blumberg, 1994; Gath, 1985; Glover and Glover, 1996; Kupperman, Golberg, Nease and Washington, 1999; Pueschel, 1991). When considering these common depictions or constructions of people with Down syndrome, it is not surprising that the birth of a child with Down syndrome has often been described as a 'tragic instance' (Berube, 1996: 25) and greeted with feelings of loss and disappointment. While not discounting that there are biological differences in a person with Down syndrome, the development of the biomedical, historical, and cultural forms of discourse about Down syndrome, and parenting children with Down syndrome appears to be inordinately skewed to mean pathology and negative experience.

149

These dominant depictions of Down syndrome currently support the genetic testing programs for Down syndrome that continue to expand and develop (Blumberg, 1994; Elkins and Brown, 1995; Glover and Glover, 1996; Williams, 1995). As prenatal diagnosis becomes more common, an increasing number of prospective parents are faced with difficult decisions. To date, there are no specific regional statistics regarding the incidence of elective abortion following the prenatal diagnosis of Down syndrome. However, Palmer et al. (1993), Blumberg (1994), Berube (1996), and Glover and Glover (1996) state that most women, faced with the diagnosis of Down syndrome, choose to terminate the pregnancy. This situation seems reasonable considering that the dominant view of Down syndrome is one of ongoing burden.

However, the engrained cultural depictions of Down syndrome and parenting a child with Down syndrome are starting to be challenged. At the same time as genetic testing is becoming more prevalent, increasing numbers of people are starting to question the current dominant constructions of Down syndrome and parenting a child with Down syndrome. More people are talking about ways in which people with Down syndrome are of value to society and how they enrich people's lives. The study to be shared in this chapter is about continuing to open spaces for more appreciative voices to be heard in the cultural dialogues on parenting a child with Down syndrome.

This study was conducted using a social constructionist perspective where two primary premises hold:

(1) the way we converse with others is a key factor in the meanings we construct;
(2) and that these meanings are continually negotiable.

Coming from this perspective, the prevailing views on Down syndrome and parenting children with Down syndrome are regarded as dominant cultural portrayals or constructions and these dominant constructions are considered negotiable.

Significance of study

This study is not about denying the fears, struggles and difficulties parents may face raising a child with Down syndrome. The importance of this study rests in the researcher's fear that the increase in genetic testing represents an increase in negative perceptions of persons with Down syndrome within our society. These negative perceptions, along with the increased availability and subsequent use of genetic testing, have created a situation where foetuses with Down syndrome have become particularly vulnerable. Growing numbers of prospective parents are faced with making life or death decisions regarding a foetus with Down syndrome. This study is not about judging prospective parents' final decisions as right or wrong since each genetic decision is unique and influenced by multiple factors. However, for this critical decision-making process, parents deserve a broad picture of what it is like to share one's life with a child with Down syndrome from birth to adulthood so that prospective parents' decisions are well informed.

Health professionals (doctors, specialists, genetic counsellors, and/or counsellors) play an important role in supporting prospective parents in this deliberative process by providing a wide range of considerations, perspectives and options. The meanings and images created about parenting a child with Down syndrome from the appreciative dialogues contained in this chapter are intended to add breadth to factors considered by prospective parents, and the health care professionals who assist them, in making decisions about the future of foetuses with Down syndrome.

Philosophical stance

The perspective that informed this study derives directly from the researcher's personal experience and philosophical stance. The researcher is the sister of a person with Down syndrome and was married for 21 years into a First Nation's (aboriginal, native American) culture. These experiences, along with those of being a mother, teacher and counsellor, all profoundly contributed to the researcher's choice of topic and methodology. In addition to these personal experiences, beliefs about knowledge and how it is used in society gave some impetus to the study. The researcher worked from the premise that it is important to challenge taken-for-granted assumptions about 'reality', thereby allowing other possible ways of understanding to emerge.

Methodology

Social constructionist inquiry

Today there are a wide range of active inquiries devoted to understanding the construction of self and world. One of these ways is called the social constructionist movement, and this paper reflects this approach. A social constructionist inquiry focuses on social approach. According to Gergen (1994), renowned scholar of social construction, there are several important assumptions that are made by a social constructionist science:

• The terms by which we account for the world and ourselves are not dictated by the stipulated objects of such accounts.

- We understand the world and ourselves within the context of relation-ship.
- Language derives its significance in human affairs from the way in which it functions within patterns of relationship. All societies/cultures develop forms of discourse for carrying out their collective lives. People in relationships (societies, cultures) use forms of discourse to construct and share meanings.
- Using forms of discourse people move towards collective agreements on what they consider to be real, rational and right (best fit). Meanings are continually negotiated until people find something that works for them.
- In language there are taken-for-granted patterns, repetitiveness, and engrained patterns. Thus language used in local ways may exclude other experiences.

By using a social constructionist framework, this study invites reflection on our society's taken-for-granted assumptions regarding Down syndrome. Gergen (1999) describes the dangers inherent in the solidification of any given way of constructing the world. He states:

> It is essential to set in motion processes of reflexive deliberation, processes which call attention to the historically and culturally situated character of the taken-for-granted world, which reflect on their potentials for suppression, and open a space for other dialogues of the culture. . . Reflexive deliberation has been, and continues to be, a significant form of scholarship within the constructionist frame.
>
> (1999: 5)

This study used the processes of reflexive deliberation and focused on the experiences parents appreciate about parenting a child with Down syndrome, experiences that have been largely excluded from the dominant discourses about parenting a child with Down syndrome from birth to adult-hood.

Appreciative inquiry

An application of social constructionist thought used in this research is termed 'appreciative inquiry'. Appreciative inquiry, according to Gergen (1982, 1990), treats social and psychological reality as a product of the moment, open to continuous reconstruction. Cooperrider and Srivastva (1987) contend that looking at the problems in inquiry reduces the possi-bility of generating new images of social reality, new theory that might help transcend current social forms. Appreciative inquiry is considered a process of joining together in a common cause to find hidden hopes and strengths. In the research reported here the focus of such an inquiry was specifically parenting a child with Down syndrome.

By choosing an appreciative approach, asking questions, engaging in conversations and then analysing the transcribed conversations, the researcher acknowledges being part of these constructions of appreciation presented here. This study was not a case of discovering appreciation, but rather by engaging parents in conversations about appreciation, the participants and the researcher actively constructed these meanings of appreciation together.

Research question

What experiences are appreciated by primary parent caregivers living with a child with Down syndrome from birth to adulthood?

Dimensions of the sample

Participants were recruited for this study using purposive sampling, a procedure where people are intentionally sought because they meet the criteria established for inclusion in the research. Two people working directly with adults with Down syndrome suggested parents who met the inclusion criteria – which were that they were a primary parent caregiver and had a child with Down syndrome over the age of 18. Nine parents, six mothers and three fathers, of six adult children with Down syndrome ranging in age from 18 to 40 years were ultimately interviewed. Each parent or set of parents was interviewed twice, the initial interview and then a second interview to clarify and validate data analysis. Each interview took from one to two hours to complete.

Discussion

Through conversations between the researcher and the participating parents, and through research analysis validated later by the participants, three central themes were constructed regarding experiences appreciated by parents of children with Down syndrome spanning the time from birth to adulthood:

Theme one: Awareness and acceptance – a reconstruction process;
Theme two: Child as teacher;
Theme three: Caregiver appreciation.

Theme one – Awareness and acceptance

The first theme looked at the reconstructing process parents appeared to go through after they became aware that their child had been labelled with Down syndrome. Upon being told their child had Down syndrome, parents struggled with intense feelings, confusion, and disbelief. This was not a joy-filled celebration time for parents where they immediately expressed appreciation for this child with Down syndrome. Conversations about appreciation could not have been constructed with these parents at this time.

However, as they began to acknowledge that this child was not who they had previously imagined, not considered normal or perfect, a process of reconstruction or acceptance began. Parents referred to this process as 'a gradual process', 'totally revamp(ing)', 'chang(ing) your ideas on', 'restructur(ing) your thoughts', 'readapt(ing), refocus(ing), rechang(ing)'. Repeatedly parents talked about a process for them where they 'learned to accept' this child with Down syndrome for who he or she was. The word 'accept' appeared repeatedly as parents, each parent in his or her way, eventually said 'yes' to this child. In the WorldWide Webster Dictionary the word *appreciate* means 'to grasp the nature, worth, quality or significance of, to judge with heightened perception or understanding, and to recognize with gratitude'. In order for parents to be thankful for or recognize the worth of their child with Down syndrome they appeared to have to let go of the concepts of the perfect or normal child and to accept this different child, this child labelled with Down syndrome:

> All the expectations you have for this normal child go out the window. You have to totally revamp . . . you have to totally restructure your thoughts.

> You have to take your own ideals of what you thought life was going to be, this perfect child you're going to have and you don't, and all of a sudden you've got one you've got to change your ideas on . . . you have to learn to accept this.

> My son fits where he fits. I learned to readapt, refocus and rechange.

> I've learned to accept him . . . as much as I never would have said this when he was born – I wouldn't change having him.

This process was unique for each parent. Nonetheless, parents consistently responded with descriptions of how they gradually began accepting their child with Down syndrome.

Theme two – Child as teacher

Throughout the interviews, parents shared their appreciation for their children as teachers. Parents used words like 'I've learned', 'he shows us', 'he turned my thoughts', 'he let me see that', 'he's taught us a lot', 'he's there to teach you', 'you learn', 'he made us appreciate', 'it's been rather enlightening', 'I've been able to experience whereas I wouldn't of'. The parents spoke of how their lives had shifted because they took something from their experiences with their children with Down syndrome and learned from them. Parents talked about learning more about humility, patience, loving, compassion, forgiveness, valuing small things, optimism, acceptance of themselves and others, determination, kindness, family relationships, judgements, and selfishness. One parent stated how she appreciated her shift from patterns of what she considered selfishness and pride to a place of more humility as she experienced life with her child with Down syndrome:

> I don't think I'd be the person I am today. I think I'd be more selfish and I certainly am more humble. Before our son was born I was quite proud of myself, thinking that a lot of things I did were superior to other people . . . and he just let me see that . . . everybody is the same and nobody is superior to anybody else and then I saw people in a different way . . . I wasn't so judgmental about them.

When people think of teachers, it is not likely that someone with Down syndrome comes to mind. The idea of someone with Down syndrome as a wise teacher is a different understanding, one this study adds to the discourse about people with Down syndrome:

> He's taught me lots. I've taught him lots but he's also taught me more . . . You will learn something from his downfalls, you will learn from his joys, you will learn from everything but at a greater scale than you would a normal child . . . he's taught me more at a deeper level . . . He's taught me to look at life differently, very, very differently. You see things you wouldn't see before.

> I think some of these people teach us a lot more than any teacher ever taught.

Theme three – Caregiver appreciation

The third theme focused on the role of caregiving and what parents appreciated about that role. The term caregiver as used in this study is based on the idea of family-based care through a lifetime (Heller, 1993). For some parents the care was all encompassing and these caregivers explained that the care of their adult child with Down syndrome gave their lives meaning and purpose. These parents were totally immersed in caregiving from which they derived a great deal of pleasure:

> Separate me from my son and you'd destroy me.

> You can't just sit down and die because we've got our son to keep us moving, keep us busy.

> I didn't have a job so this became my focus . . . this became an enchantment for me . . . I had a focus, I felt worthwhile.

For other parents the role of caregiver was not so encompassing. However, regardless of how much emphasis parents put on the role of caregiver, all parents appeared to appreciate becoming advocates for their children, working hard with and for them and then watching their children accomplish things they never thought were possible. They appeared to appreciate different aspects of their own hard work and how it was connected to their children's accomplishments.

> I remember just how rewarding his accomplishments were . . . every little accomplishment is absolutely huge . . . that you work so hard towards, that he works so hard towards . . . going through school and then advancing to college . . . I basically was told that he would probably never read and he wouldn't write . . . everything was exceeded . . . and I guess the last eventful thing was him getting married . . . I in all expectations probably didn't expect to happen . . . you know you just keep getting rewards year after year and you know its quite amazing.

This research is consistent with Van Riper's (1999) findings to date, which indicate that

> while the birth of a child with Down syndrome involves a 'change of plans' for families, it does not have to be a negative experience. In fact, for many families, it is a positive, growth producing experience.
>
> (1999: 3)

Parents in this study indicated that their lives have been enhanced by the experiences involved in raising a child with Down syndrome from birth to adulthood. Many parents said they would now never wish for a child labelled normal, that their lives were somehow better as a result of these experiences. These findings agree with Gath's (1985) where a notable number of families have found their lives were enhanced by what they originally thought was going to be an unbearable burden. As well, this study adds parents' voices to academic literature; voices Goodey (1991) says have been seldom heard.

Implications for further research and practice

This research indicates that for some families at least, having a child with Down syndrome is not the negative experience so often depicted. Clearly, however, there is much to be done in educating the general public and health professionals about the positive aspects of having a family member with Down syndrome. Portrayals of people with Down syndrome need to be expanded and changed to include the positive elements identified in this study as well as in others. More research that focuses on resilience, adaptation, and the positive aspects of living with a person with Down syndrome needs to be undertaken.

Parents involved in this study gave birth to their children with Down syndrome 20 to 40 years ago. Although support for parents and their children with Down syndrome has increased dramatically since that time, negative depictions of Down syndrome persist. With the increasing opportunities for genetic testing, many prospective parents are now faced with difficult decisions, decisions prospective parents were never faced with in the past. Research to date suggests that prospective parents need to be provided with:

- A clearer understanding of genetic testing procedures and test results.
- All of the options available to them if a prenatal diagnosis is positive.
- More opportunities for counselling and support (Blumberg, 1994; Elkins, Stovall, Wilroy, and Dacus, 1986; Helm, Miranda, and Chedd, 1998; Pueschel, 1991; Spudich, 1992; Statham and Green, 1993; Stein 1997).

Conclusion

This study offers a 'glass half full' perspective. In conversations with the researcher, parents shared a wide range of experiences they appreciated having lived with a child with Down syndrome from birth to adulthood. This research is about how parents have said 'yes' to a child when the child was born with Down syndrome, how they have constructed concepts of appreciation even though the dominant articulations about Down syndrome are rooted in pathology and deficit. This research gives another perspective, that a child with Down syndrome can be celebrated and enjoyed. By constructing an appreciative perspective with the researcher, parents have shared elements of human possibilities that might have otherwise gone unheard.

References

Berube M (1996) Life As We Know It. Toronto: Random House of Canada Limited.

Blumberg L (1994) The politics of prenatal testing and selective abortion. Sexuality and Disability 12: 135-53.

Cooperrider DL, Srivastva S (1987) Appreciative inquiry in organizational life. In Woodman R, Pasmore W (Eds) Research in Organization Change and Development: Vol 1. Greenwich, CT: JAI Press. pp 129-69.

Elkins TE, Brown D (1995) Ethical concerns and future directions in maternal screening for Down syndrome. Women's Health Issues 5: 15-20.

Elkins TE, Stovall TG, Wilroy S, Dacus JV (1986) Attitudes of mothers of children with Down syndrome concerning amniocentesis, abortion, and prenatal genetic counseling techniques. Obstetrics and Gynecology 68: 181-4.

Gath A (1985) Parental reactions to loss and disappointment: the diagnosis of Down's syndrome. Developmental Medicine and Child Neurology 27: 392-400.

Gergen K (1982) Toward Transformation in Social Knowledge. New York: Springer-Verlag.

Gergen K (1990) Affect and organization in postmodern society. In Srivastva S, Cooperrider DL (Eds) Appreciative Management and Leadership. San Francisco: Jossey-Bass. pp 153-74.

Gergen K (1994) Realities and Relationships. Cambridge: Harvard University Press.

Gergen K (1999) Social psychology as social construction: the emerging vision. In McGarty C, Haslam A (Eds) The Message of Social Psychology: Perspectives on Mind in Society. Oxford: Blackwell. Available on-line: http://www.swarthmore.edu/SocSci/kgergen1/text1.html.

Glover NM, Glover SJ (1996) Ethical and legal issues regarding selective abortion of fetuses with Down syndrome. Mental Retardation 34(4): 207-14.

Goodey CF (1991) Living in the Real World. London: Twenty-One Press.

Heller T (1993) Aging caregivers of persons with developmental disabilities: changes in burden and placement desire. In Roberto KA (Ed) The Elderly Caregiver. Newbury Park, CA: Sage Publications. pp 21-39.

Helm DT, Miranda S, Chedd NA (1998) Prenatal diagnosis of Down syndrome: mothers' reflections on supports needed from diagnosis to birth. Mental Retardation 36: 55-61.

Kupperman M, Golberg JD, Nease RF, Washington A (1999) Who should be offered prenatal diagnosis? The 35-year-old question. American Journal of Public Health 89: 160-64.

McDonough P (1990) Congenital disability and medical research: the development of amniocentesis. Women and Health 16: 137-53.

Palmer S, Spencer J, Kushnick T, Wiley J, Bowyer S (1993) Follow up survey of pregnancies with diagnoses of chromosomal abnormality. Journal of Genetic Counseling 2: 139-52.

Pueschel SM (1991) Ethical considerations relating to prenatal diagnosis to foetuses with Down syndrome. Mental Retardation 29: 185-90.

Spudich H (1992) Looking for Answers, Finding More Questions: Report on the Vancouver Workshop on Bioethical Issues. Brussels: International League of Societies for Persons with Mental Handicap.

Statham H, Green J (1993) Serum screening for Down's syndrome: some women's experiences. British Medical Journal 307: 174-6.

Stein MT (1997) Responding to parental concerns after a prenatal diagnosis of Trisomy 21. Journal of Developmental and Behavioural Pediatrics 18: 42-6.

Stratford B (1991) Human rights and equal opportunities for people with mental handicap - with particular reference to Down Syndrome. International Journal of Disability, Development and Education 38: 3-13.

Williams P (1995) Should we prevent Down's syndrome? British Journal of Learning Disabilities 23: 46-9.

Van Riper M (1999) Living with Down syndrome: the family experience. Down Syndrome Quarterly 4: 1-7.

Chapter 13
Multiple perspectives of family life

MONICA CUSKELLY, ANNE JOBLING, DAVID CHANT, ANNA
BOWER AND ALAN HAYES

Changes in community attitudes and social policy have meant that the majority
of children with a disability now reside with their family (Hayes, 1994). This is
widely accepted as a positive change, yet it must be acknowledged that it has
brought with it the potential to increase the day-to-day stresses experienced by
family members. A feature of studies of family functioning has been the focus
on negative outcomes for families, with many studies seeking only to identify
the ways in which these families are doing less well than their counterparts
where all children are developing typically (Crnic, 1990).

Although much has been written about mothers' functioning when one
child has a disability, other family members have been relatively ignored.
Families are complex systems so it can be difficult to capture a good picture
of how they function, and certainly this will not be possible if only one
member's views are sought. Fathers, in particular, are a neglected source of
information in studies of family functioning. The few studies that do include
fathers make it clear that fathers' views and experiences differ in important
ways from those of mothers. It is therefore necessary that every effort is
made to include their perspectives when a picture of family functioning is
sought. The brothers and sisters of a child with a disability have received
more attention than fathers. However, as with other family-focused research,
much of this work has been with groups comprising a wide variety of
disabling conditions.

Research designs that group all families with a child with a disability
together, irrespective of the nature of the disability, acknowledge the
commonality of the experience of having a child with a disability – the
additional financial costs, the worries about the child's social acceptance, the
concerns about the impact on brothers and sisters, the doubts about finding
an accepting and helpful school and later a workplace that offers respect and
meaningful employment. There are, however, limitations to this approach of

grouping all families together that have been discussed at some length (see, Cuskelly, 1999; Lobato, Faust and Spirito, 1988). The disadvantages would appear to outweigh the advantages as an understanding of the shared experiences can be achieved by an accumulation of evidence from different groups, while the problems that arise when different disabilities are treated as homogeneous cannot be overcome.

Three studies of families of a school-aged child with Down syndrome are presented below. All had a focus on family coping rather than failure, all were open to the possibility of positive outcomes for family members and all attempted to develop our understanding of some of the supports and constraints under which families operate. Each study focused on a different subset of the family. The first investigated mothers' perspectives of their families while the second investigated mothers' and fathers' feelings of stress. The third study investigated family and child variables that support a good relationship between children with Down syndrome and their brothers/sisters.

Different methodologies were employed across the studies, although all included a comparison group to allow a contrast with families in which all children were typically developing. This is a common approach to examining family life when there is a child with a disability; however, it has an inherent danger as it carries with it the expectation that any differences are caused by the disability when this, in fact, may not be the case. The first study used a qualitative method, which allowed an immensely rich data set to be collected, with the results providing an heuristic which will be helpful to other researchers interested in extending our understanding of maternal perspectives. The approach was based in grounded theory, where understanding is created from the emerging data. The other two studies used a quantitative approach. Both utilized semi-structured interviewing as the data collection method and both collected information about areas of possible strength as well as about possible difficulties. The latter two studies included two-parent families only. Our decision here was a pragmatic one rather than reflecting any philosophical position – to add another variable to the mix would have made our data very difficult to interpret.

Study 1: Mothers' experiences of mothering

Data collection

Open and semi-structured interviews were used in this study so that mothers could respond to the issues in their own way, a process which facilitates theory development. Mothers had a great deal of control in determining the direction of the interview and their responses contained highly personal content of individual significance. The data reported here were generally collected in one long interview by a researcher with experience of working with parents. All interviews were recorded for later transcription and analysis.

Three groups were included in this study (mothers of a child with Down syndrome, mothers of a child with spina bifida, and mothers whose children were all developing typically), however only the data from the mothers of a child with Down syndrome and those whose children were developing typically will be reported here. Twenty mothers of a child with Down syndrome between the ages of 8 and 13 years (11 girls and nine boys) with a sibling within approximately 1 to 3 years were interviewed. Forty comparison mothers with children in the same age ranges also participated. This age range was selected as middle childhood has been a neglected period in research. All children with Down syndrome were functioning in the moderate to severe range of intellectual disability and all enjoyed good health. Comparison families were selected to match the focus families as closely as possible with first priority given to the variables of age, gender, and position in family for both children. Second priority was given to parental education, occupation and age. Two mothers of a child with Down syndrome were permanently separated from their husbands at the time of interview, one comparison mother was divorced and another was living in a de facto relationship.

Results

One hundred and ten categories were identified from the data after transcription. The six categories which arose most frequently are listed below. They are not in order of frequency but have been grouped thematically. Excerpts from the transcripts (names changed) are included to illustrate the variety of ways in which mothers expressed their concerns. Transcripts are not attributed but those included here come from a number of different mothers all who have a child with Down syndrome.

Family cohesion

The concept of family cohesion, often expressed as family harmony and getting along with one another, was a recurrent theme. One of the most important indicators used by mothers to judge their success as mothers appeared to be whether they believed that they had achieved cohesion among family members. The mothers described family cohesion in several ways, ranging from spousal support, the inclusion of members of the extended family, to simply joint family activity and enjoyment. It is apparent that this unity represents a strength within families and appeared to represent security and stability for mothers.

> maybe it's the whole . . . the family as a unit in the sense that it has made us all closer and stronger. I mean we all stick together, you know . . . and we'll all be there for each other, because we've had to help each other through.

Sibling relationships

Mothers perceived supportive and harmonious sibling relationships as evidence of successful mothering. Some mothers desired a good sibling relationship as they anticipated that siblings would continue to care for the child with disability, once the parents, and specifically the mother, could no longer do so. Key terms they used in their accounts of their children's positive social behaviour towards one another included: 'awareness of needs', 'being responsible', 'accepting' and 'protective'.

> I've got to say . . . she is still a child and there are times when she lets that all hang loose, but uhm . . . you know . . . socially when we are out anywhere, she is very aware of Kylie's needs and fully accepting.

> . . . but at school the headmaster said that Daniel and Tim are very close and very protective of one another.

Father/child relationship

The relationships fathers have with their children significantly influence mothers' ideas about family functioning and their mothering role. Positive relationships between fathers and their children signal family cohesion to mothers, strongly contributing to mothers' perception of success in their mothering role. It may be assumed that stable and positive relationships between fathers and children enhance mothers' feelings of resilience, whereas dysfunctional or nonexistent relationships may increase the chances of mothers feeling vulnerable.

Although mothers were encouraged to talk about the entire range of family relationships, some mothers clearly avoided talking about the fathers of their children. The mothers who did discuss these relationships can be divided into two groups: those who proudly reported solid and functional relationships; and those who indicated that they were not comfortable with the existing relationship their partners had with their children. Consider the following positive statements:

> . . . they are so fond of him and he is terrific with them.

> . . . they get on absolutely wonderful together . . . her handsome father . . . well . . . she absolutely adores her father.

The following example describes a more difficult father–child relationship:

> He is not particularly patient with Cecilia, he thinks she should really be able to do it, and once told not to do something, she should understand not to do it . . . He finds her very irritating . . . she couldn't say what she wanted and he would lose his patience.

Interestingly, most of the mothers who raised the father–child relationship issue focused on the father's relationship with the child with a disability, indicating that this relationship perhaps is at higher risk. The ideas these mothers presented suggest that they desire a close father–child relationship, but in its absence, they tend to take on a very protective role of the child or children whom they perceive as not being adequately understood by their father.

The crucial issue for mothers appears to be whether their partners' interactions with their child(ren) meet their own values and expectations. The responses of the mothers in this study suggest that met expectations tend to promote feelings of resilience, whereas differences in values and expectations are more likely to result in mothers' feelings of vulnerability.

Hopes and expectations

The hopes and expectations mothers hold for their family, but more specifically for the children, were a recurring theme in their discussions. Mothers tended to express their hopes in tentative ways, allowing ample margins for changes in children's individual development and in family life. Conversely, expectations tended to be expressed in more definite ways and appeared to be influenced by mothers' own childhood and family experiences and in many instances by their partners' views. Mothers' expectations were expressed as long-term objectives for child and family development, and these tended to be linked with perceptions of successful mothering.

Mothers who have a child with Down syndrome tended to have a strong focus on independence for their children, but specifically for their child with an intellectual disability. While some mothers expressed their concerns in terms of hope for independence, others appeared to have more definite expectations for this to occur, although a number of mothers expressed reservations about their child's safety.

> You know I guess my dreams are that he will be an independent, active part of the community, were it be a fairly small, isolated community or a large extended city type community.

> . . . well, I was driving at the weekend and there were two bouncing young girls on a traffic island in the middle of the road waiting for the traffic to go or for the lights to change. And they were really pretty and I said . . . that is how Marsha is going to look like. They had a perm in their hair. They were dressed up for their lunchtime. They were going out somewhere, and I said . . . isn't that nice, you know . . . and I saw Marsha doing that.

> Kylie, I'm finding I've always said that my plans for her were to become independent, and I'm probably . . . they still are, but the older she gets, the more frightened

I get about her being taken advantage of. And that makes me want to pull her close again . . . yes . . . and I know it's wrong, so this is an issue I am grappling with . . . Uhm . . . and I mean as far as her being capable of living an independent life, I am all for that, and I would like to encourage that every inch of the way . . . uhm . . . but as I say, that is my one fear.

Vulnerability

Vulnerability is generally discussed in terms of being the opposite of resilience. However, people cannot be simply categorized as either vulnerable or resilient, because most people experience both states at different times of their lives. It is important to ascertain not only mothers' feelings of resilience, but also the feelings of vulnerability they may experience in the course of mothering. While resilience indicates a person's ability to cope with a stressful situation, vulnerability implies exposure to uncertainty and a likely decrease in the ability to cope effectively, to feel in control and capable of accepting challenge and commitment.

If you don't have a child . . . uhm . . . an intellectually disabled child of your own, it's very easy to hypothesize, but when it becomes your child, the issues just change . . . totally! I find . . . as we go on, we come face to face with each issue. What once would have been an easy solution isn't any more, because it's your child.

Resilience/hardiness

Personal resilience is a significant feature of coping and appeared to be an important resource for the mothers in this study. It is defined as the ability to seek and accept family support (Bernheimer, Gallimore and Weisner, 1990), the ability to acknowledge and accept demanding situations, the ability to be assertive in both thought and action and the potential to benefit from spiritual and philosophical support. The related construct of hardiness, defined by Kobasa (1979) as the ability to accept challenge, take control and sustain commitment, also arose many times in the mothers' conversations.

Mothers spoke of a number of mechanisms which supported them: of most importance, however, were (a) family support and (b) certain spiritual or philosophical beliefs, findings which are reflected elsewhere (e.g. Weisner, Beizer and Stolze, 1991).

Resilience and family support

The importance of family support is widely documented in the literature on family and disability (e.g. Fewell, 1986; Gartner, Lipsky and Turnbull, 1991; Hayes, 1994; Shapiro, 1989), and is generally acknowledged to be a key coping resource (Beresford, 1994). The following provides some insight into mothers' perceptions about family support and its link to resilience.

. . . well I suppose just as a unit you are sort of a lot more stronger. I mean you know, I think after Camilla being born I don't think sort of anything could really happen, that would sort of shake anything. You just cope with it, because you have to, and you stick together, because you know the buck stops right here, and together you just muddle your way through. It's been like that now for 13 years.

Resilience and spiritual/philosophical beliefs

Spiritual or philosophical support systems were also commonly identified as a crucial source of personal support in this study as in others (e.g. Fewell, 1986). A number of mothers with a child with disability in this study identified religious faith as a coping resource, resulting in personal resilience, while, alternatively, some mothers identified non-spiritual but personal philosophical attitudes as a strength which promoted personal resilience.

I will say this too . . . when Charlotte was born she was . . . uhm . . . like my mission in life I was put on this earth to do my very best for this child, and it made me strong.

Conclusion

Few differences were found between mothers of typically developing children and mothers of a child with Down syndrome. Having a child with a disability may have bought some issues into sharper relief (e.g. family relationships, development of independence); however, the aspects of mothering given most prominence were similar across the groups. Mothers' perceptions and ideas about fathers' relationships with their children were clearly of importance: however, it is necessary to remember that mothers' perceptions may differ considerably from fathers' own perceptions of their involvement with their children.

Study 2: Stress in mothers and fathers

Clearly, parental stress is an indicator of one aspect of family functioning and there are a number of studies which have identified this as a substantial problem for parents of a child with a disability (e.g. Fuller and Rankin, 1994; Dyson, 1997). It is also identified as an important issue by parents whose children have no developmental delay. The present report focuses on stress and on family variables which may act to ameliorate or compound the stress experienced by parents.

Data collection

Sixty-four families who had a child with Down syndrome between the two age bands of 4 years 6 months to 8 years 6 months and 12 years 6 months to

16 years 6 months participated in the study, along with 89 comparison families who also had a child in one of these age bands. There were no significant differences between the groups on the demographic variables of number of children, age of youngest child, or occupational status.

All families were seen on two occasions by two interviewers (one interviewed the mother and the other the father). In contrast to the study described above, the interviews for this study were conducted using a series of questionnaires. All questions were presented by the interviewers and discussed if necessary before a response was recorded. The data from five questionnaires are included in the analyses reported here.

Stress was measured using the Parenting Stress Index (PSI: Abidin, 1990). The PSI provides information on two domains of parenting stress – parent and child characteristics. The parent scale comprises seven subscales: Depression; Sense of Competence; Parental Attachment; Relationship with Spouse; Social Isolation; Parental Health; and Restriction of Role. The child scale has six subscales: Adaptability; Demandingness; Child Mood; Distractibility/Hyperactivity; Acceptability; and Child Reinforces the Parent. In addition a total score can be derived. High scores are indicative of family dysfunction (Abidin, 1990) and normative information is available.

The experience of stress may be ameliorated by support (Gartner et al., 1991; Shapiro, 1989), which may take a number of forms. The Family Support Scale (FSS: Dunst, Trivette and Hamby, 1994) was developed to identify sources of support used by individual families in the preceding six months and to assess the perceived helpfulness of these supports. The sources of support include members within the immediate family, members of the extended family, friends, and community services.

The issue of within-family support is particularly interesting and two additional measures were included in this study. All families have multiple areas of responsibilities and so cooperation from children with one area of common responsibility – household tasks – can ease the parental burden. The Children's Task Participation Scale (Bird and Ratcliff, 1990) provides information on the division of parental responsibility and children's assumption of personal and domestic responsibilities. In its initial form it contained 17 items: however, an additional five items were added to reflect common tasks required of children (ironing, putting out the rubbish, supervising homework of siblings, maintaining personal hygiene, and outdoor tasks). The contributions of all children (excluding infants and toddlers) were included in this analysis.

There are now several studies which have found that the daily hassles experienced in family life are more stressful for parents than are 'larger' but infrequent stressor events (e.g. Ruffin, 1993). The Daily Parenting Hassles Questionnaire (Crnic and Greenberg, 1990) assesses parents' experience of a range of typical, often irritating, child behaviours, such as nagging, whining or complaining. It yields two scales – frequency and intensity – which are highly correlated. The absence of high levels of daily hassles was interpreted for this study as an indicator of within-family support.

Results

Table 13.1 shows the average score for each subscale of the PSI for each group and also contains the average of the normative sample. On two of the subscales in the parenting domain – *Depression* and *Sense of Competence* – there was a significant difference between the groups, with parents of a child with Down syndrome reporting more stress than comparison parents. The total score is also significantly higher for these parents. Clearly, however, the average levels of stress for the parents of a child with Down syndrome are well within the average range. Some significant differences occurred between mothers and fathers as noted in Table 13.1. On all but one of the identified scales (*Social Isolation*) mothers reported finding their parenting role more stressful than did fathers. Fathers, however, felt more socially isolated.

On all of the subscales on the Child Domain, with the exception of the subscale *Reinforces Parent*, there were significant differences between the groups. On most scales, parents of a child with Down syndrome reported more stress than comparison parents. Only on the subscale *Acceptability* are parents of a child with Down syndrome outside the average range for the norming group. The intent of this scale is to pick up discrepancies between the expected child and the real child and the assumption is that such discrepancies produce stress. Although these discrepancies exist, their impact on the experience of stress may be less than expected, at least by the time the child is of the ages included here. Mothers of a child with Down syndrome reported that they found their child to be *more* reinforcing than did mothers of typically developing children and parents of a child with Down syndrome reported few problems associated with the child's mood.

Both mothers and fathers of a child with Down syndrome reported they had received more support from family and community than comparison parents (FSS). The measure which collected information about children's participation in tasks around the home showed no differences between the groups. Children in each group gave as much (or as little) assistance around the home as each other and this was true across the four subscales. There were no differences between families who had a child with Down syndrome and comparison families in either the frequency of hassles or in the intensity of these common problems. The role of family support in the experience of stress was tested using a regression analysis. Only the *Social Isolation* subscale of the PSI was found to be influenced by the perceived level of social support provided to the family.

Table 13.1 Mean Parenting Stress Index scores for parents of a child with Down syndrome and comparison parents, and normative information (standard deviation)

	Parents of a child with Down syndrome	Comparison parents	Norms	
Parent Depression*#	21.14	18.83	20.3	(5.5)
Parent Attachment	13.74	13.73	12.7	(3.2)
Restriction of Role#	17.48	16.79	18.9	(5.3)
Sense of Competence*#	31.80	27.77	29.1	(6.0)
Social Isolation#	13.51	12.78	12.6	(3.7)
Relationship with Spouse#	17.09	16.11	16.9	(5.1)
Parental Health#	12.26	11.73	16.9	(3.4)
Parent Domain Score*#	126.98	117.76	123.1	(24.4)
Child Adaptability*	28.17	25.02	24.9	(5.7)
Child Acceptability*	19.03	12.66	12.6	(3.5)
Child Demands*#	22.55	18.74	18.3	(4.6)
Child Mood*	10.07	11.27	9.7	(2.9)
Child Distractability*	25.88	22.51	24.7	(4.8)
Reinforces Parent (interaction)	10.94	11.66	9.4	(2.9)
Child Domain Score*	116.60	101.97	99.7	(18.8)

* A statistically significant difference between parents of a child with Down syndrome and comparison parents.
# A statistically significant difference between mothers and fathers.

Conclusions

It is clear from the results reported here that in many ways the families with a child with Down syndrome are more like other families than they are different. This does not mean that some families do not experience deep distress about some aspects of their child's life but also it is inappropriate to assume that having a child with Down syndrome inevitably produces stress when the majority of families demonstrate healthy functioning in their day-to-day lives.

Study 3: Sibling relationships

As shown above, the relationship between the child with Down syndrome and his or her brothers or sisters is an issue of great importance to mothers of these children. In this they reflect a concern of most mothers who see one of their prime responsibilities to be the development of a positive relationship between their children (Bower, 1997).

Recent studies which have examined this issue have generally found that mothers' reports of the sibling relationship are either very similar across groups or that the sibling of the child with the disability behaves in a more positive way than do comparison children (Bagenholm and Gillberg, 1991; McHale and Gamble, 1989; McHale, Sloan and Simeonsson, 1986). Children's reports reflect the same finding – brothers and sisters of a child with a disability report that they behave in ways that are similar to or more positive than comparison children in their dealing with their sibling (McHale et al., 1986; McHale and Gamble, 1987). Few researchers have attempted to determine what contributes to these good relationships.

Data collection

Each family of a child with Down syndrome was matched to a comparison family at the individual level to ensure that any differences between groups would not be due to 'social address' variables. Matching was at both the level of the child (age, sex, position in family, position relative to other child) and the family (number in the family, father's occupation). The focus sibling was between the ages of 7 and 14 years and the other child, including the child with Down syndrome, was between the ages of 5 years 6 months and 18 years. All sibling pairs were no more than four years apart and were the nearest in age.

Mothers, fathers and the sibling who was the focus of the study completed a questionnaire which asked how often certain behaviours were displayed by the focus sibling. The Sibling Inventory of Behaviour (Schaefer and Edgerton, 1981) contains questions about behaviours which are positive and those which are negative. Composite scores (positive and negative) were used for the analyses reported here. Factor analysis and measures of internal reliability supported this use of the data. As one-off reports of behaviour may be unreliable and as it is possible that children's reports are unduly influenced by recent occurrences, we included four telephone calls in order to provide an accuracy check on the information provided by the siblings. Information was collected about the interaction between the sibling pair on the day of the telephone call.

Parental satisfaction with their partner's parenting was assessed using a questionnaire developed for this study. Each parent was asked a series of questions about such issues as time spent with the children, perceived favouritism, and agreement about discipline strategies. The parent–child relationship was assessed via children's reports of their daily interactions with each parent which were collected during the telephone interviews. During every call children were asked a series of questions about their interactions with their mother and father during the day of the call. For the analyses these data were averaged.

Mothers were asked to complete the General Impressions Survey (McDevitt and Carey, 1978) to provide information about temperament of the sibling pair. This instrument reflects conceptions of temperament described by Thomas and Chess (1977) and asks parents to rate their child on the nine temperament scales and also to give a rating of their child's overall 'difficultness' with respect to temperament.

Results

Mothers' and fathers' reports of the positive aspects of the sibling relationship were comparable across the two groups. However, there was a trend for the brothers and sisters of a child with Down syndrome to report themselves as being more positive in their interactions with their brother/sister than were comparison children. A similar result was found for the negative composite – there were no differences between mothers or fathers across the two groups but there was a trend for children in the comparison group to report themselves to behave more negatively towards their brother/sister than siblings of a child with Down syndrome.

When the behaviour of brothers was compared with that of sisters no sex differences were found for any of the three rater groups (mothers, fathers, children). However, boys were significantly more negative in their reports of their relationship if the other sibling was a girl. There was also a trend for boys to be less positive when their sibling partner was a girl and these trends were apparent for both groups.

Spacing (i.e. whether the sibling was younger or older than the other child) appeared to have an impact on fathers' ratings only. Fathers reported more positive behaviour when the child being rated was older than their brother/sister.

When comparisons were made across the raters no significant differences were found on the mean scores of either the positive or negative composites. In addition to there being no differences between the group averages the distributions were also similar – unlike McHale et al. (1986) we did not find a bi-modal distribution among the brothers and sisters of a child with Down syndrome. Moreover, mothers and fathers were in agreement about these aspects of their children's relationship. There was less agreement among children and their parents about negative behaviour than there was about positive behaviour.

Mothers' and children's reports of caregiving behaviour were highly correlated. Both maternal and child reports indicated that the siblings of a child with Down syndrome, and children who were older than their brother/sister, undertook more caregiving. There were 18 first-borns in the comparison children and 19 in the brothers/sisters of a child with Down syndrome. Most comparison children in the upper 25 per cent of caregiving scores were first-borns (11/13) while only four of the 14 children in this upper fourth who were the sibling of a child with Down syndrome were first-borns. Perhaps there is some aspect of sharing the load in these families. There was no sex difference related to caregiving. Children across both groups reported they did more household chores than their mothers reported the children did. As expected, older children did more than younger, however there were no sex or group differences.

There was little statistical relationship between the mothers' and fathers' reports of their satisfaction with their spouse's parenting: however, this does not tell the entire story. Many parents were very happy with their spouse's parenting and usually couples were fairly similar in their levels of contentment. There were some parents, however, who were extremely dissatisfied with their partner in this regard, while the partner was very happy with the other's performance. It was usually (but not always) mothers who expressed extremes of dissatisfaction and fathers' levels of satisfaction were higher than were mothers'.

On mothers' reports of their general impressions on difficulty the comparison group were found to be slightly easier. The difference was significant but of little practical import as it was so small (0.6 difference on a six-point scale). Girls were generally reported to be easier than boys.

There were very few significant associations between the measures discussed here and the quality of sibling relationships. The relationship did contribute some small difference to childrens' involvement in caregiving but group and spacing were more important. It was also interesting to find that fathers' satisfaction with their spouses' parenting was predicted by the positive relationships between the children.

Conclusion

The three studies reported here focused on different aspects of family functioning: one used a very different approach to the other two, but they all reached a common conclusion – the functioning of families who have a child with a disability is very similar to that of families in which all children are developing typically. This conclusion does not deny that there are differences: however, at least for the period when the child with Down syndrome is of school age, these differences would appear to be minimal. When invited to talk about a series of broad issues related to family life, mothers of a child with Down syndrome raised essentially the same concerns as comparison mothers. Family functioning with respect to sharing family tasks, the frequency and intensity of daily hassles, and the level of stress reported by both mothers and fathers were generally not substantially different between the parents of a child with Down syndrome and comparison parents. When differences were found it was clear that the parents of children with Down syndrome were within the normal range and so the differences were not of clinical significance. The sibling relationship was as positive in families with a child with Down syndrome as in comparison families.

The age of the child with Down syndrome may be an important factor in these results – certainly the birth of a child with Down syndrome can be very stressful (Shepperdson, 1988) – and it may also be the case that as the child with Down syndrome reaches adulthood this places new pressures on families. The chapter by Jobling and Cuskelly (Chapter 9, this volume) suggests that currently parents of adults with Down syndrome have much more responsibility for their adult child than is usual, and this may bring with it increased stress. The children with Down syndrome in these studies were all going to school which may act as a normalizing experience for families. It is inappropriate, however, to assume that the accommodation that these families have arrived at is a transitory phase – times are changing very rapidly in the provision of services to individuals with a disability and their families so it may well be that the families who contributed to these studies are representatives of a new wave.

The need for a concerted effort to include fathers' perspectives is made apparent by the results reported here. Two of the studies found some mothers who were very dissatisfied with their husbands' involvement with their children. Dissatisfactions of this sort can be very destructive of the family unit: however, it is unlikely that effective mechanisms to deal with or prevent this situation can be found until more is known about fathers' experiences, interpretations and strategies.

References

Adidin RR (1990) Parenting Stress Index, 3rd ed: Test Manual. Charlottesville, VA: Pediatric Psychology Press.

Bagenholm A, Gillberg C (1991) Psychosocial effects on siblings of children with autism and mental retardation: a population-based study. Journal of Mental Deficiency Research 35: 291-307.

Beresford BA (1994) Resources and strategies: how parents cope with the care of a disabled child. Journal of Child Psychology and Psychiatry 35: 171-209.

Bernheimer LP, Gallimore R, Weisner TS (1990) Ecocultural theory as a context for the individual family service plan. Journal of Early Intervention 14: 219-39.

Bird GW, Ratcliff BB (1990) Children's participation in family tasks: determinants of mothers' and fathers' reports. Human Relations 43: 865-84.

Bower A (1997) A comparative study of mothers' beliefs and ideas about mothering in families with and without disability. Unpublished doctoral dissertation, University of Queensland, Brisbane, Australia.

Crnic KA (1990) Families of children with Down syndrome: ecological contexts and characteristics. In Cicchetti D, Beeghly M (Eds) Children with Down Syndrome: A Developmental Perspective. Cambridge: Cambridge University Press. pp 399-423.

Crnic KA, Greenberg MT (1990) Minor parenting stresses with young children. Child Development 61: 1628-37.

Cuskelly M (1999) Adjustment of siblings of children with a disability: methodological issues. International Journal for the Advancement of Counselling 21: 111-24.

Dunst CJ, Trivette CM, Hamby DW (1994) Measuring social support in families with young children with disabilities. In Dunst CJ, Trivette CM (Eds) Supporting and Strengthening Families, vol 1: Methods, Strategies and Practices. Cambridge, MA: Brookline Books Inc. pp 152-60.

Dyson LL (1997) Fathers and mothers of school-age children with developmental disabilities: parental stress, family functioning, and social support. American Journal on Mental Retardation 102: 267-79.

Fewell RR (1986) A handicapped child in the family. In Fewell RR, Vadasy PF (Eds) Families of Handicapped Children: Needs and Supports Across the Lifespan. Austin: Pro-ED. pp 3-34.

Fuller GB, Rankin RE (1994) Differences in levels of parental stress among mothers of learning disabled, emotionally impaired, and regular school children. Perceptual and Motor Skills 78: 583-92.

Gartner A, Lipsky DK, Turnbull AP (1991) Supporting Families with a Child with a Disability: An International Outlook. Baltimore: Paul Brookes Pub. Co.

Hayes A (1994) Disabilities and families. In Ashman A, Elkins J (Eds) Educating Children with Special Needs (2nd ed). Sydney: Prentice Hall. pp 38-69.

Kobasa SC (1979). Stressful life events: personality and health: an inquiry into hardiness. Journal of Personality and Psychology 37: 1-11.

Lobato D, Faust D, Spirito A (1988) Examining the effects of chronic disease and disability on children's sibling relationships. Journal of Pediatric Psychology 13: 389-407.

McDevitt SC, Carey WB (1978) The measurement of temperament in three to seven year old children. Journal of Child Psychology and Psychiatry 19: 245-53.

McHale SM, Gamble WC (1987) Sibling relationships and adjustment of children with disabled brothers and sisters. In Schachter FF, Stone RK (Eds) Practical Concerns about Siblings: Bridging the Research–Practice Gap. New York: Haworth Press. pp 131-58.

McHale SM, Gamble WC (1989). Sibling relationships of children with disabled and nondisabled brothers and sisters. Developmental Psychology 25: 421-9.

McHale SM, Sloan J, Simeonsson RJ (1986) Sibling relationships with autistic, mentally retarded, and nonhandicapped brothers and sisters: a comparative study. Journal of Autism and Developmental Disorders 16: 399-414.

Ruffin CL (1993) Stress and health - little hassles vs. major life events. Australian Psychologist 28: 201-8.

Schaefer E, Edgerton M (1981) The Sibling Inventory of Behavior. Unpublished manuscript, University of North Carolina, Chapel Hill.

Shapiro J (1989) Stress, depression and support group participation in mothers of developmentally delayed children. Family Relations 38: 169-73.

Shepperdson B (1988) Growing up with Down's Syndrome. London: Cassell.

Thomas A, Chess S (1977) Temperament and Development. New York: Bruner/Mazel.

Weisner T, Beizer L, Stolze L (1991) Religion and families of children with developmental delays. American Journal on Mental Retardation 95: 647-62.

SECTION 7

VERBAL-MOTOR BEHAVIOUR

Introduction

Movement is a means through which children can explore, develop, communicate and express themselves in the world. Movement is life! However, if movement and motor skills are inefficient and ineffective this will hinder an individual's ability in everyday activities and may have a considerable negative effect on learning. Awkward walking styles, clumsiness and poor fine motor skills, which are observed as characteristics of the movement and motor skills in individuals with Down syndrome, make the motor performances of a person appear incompetent and this can reduce social acceptance in the community. Personal feelings of satisfaction and success can also be affected.

Therefore, due to the important role that movement and motor skills play in many aspects of development, the work detailed by the mainly Canadian research team of Brian Maraj, Shannon Robertson, Timothy Welsh, Daniel Weeks, Romeo Chua, Matthew Heath, Eric Roy, Dominic Simon, Harold Weinberg and Digby Elliott constitutes a significant contribution to the field of research in Down syndrome. Although theoretical in orientation, their work is endeavouring to develop an understanding of the characteristics of perceptual motor behaviour associated with Down syndrome. Are there similarities or differences in these characteristics when compared with others with intellectual disability and with children who are typically developing? Are there anatomical and/or physiological bases for the movement difficulties observed in individuals with Down syndrome? As there is much variability in the perceptual motor behaviour of individuals with Down syndrome, study replications are also essential.

The type of research described by Maraj et al. is intended to identify the reasons for the reduced motor performance of individuals with Down syndrome. Once this is established, effective strategies may be designed to ameliorate their movement problems. The knowledge gained can be used to support programs, develop interventions and raise expectations that could assist young people in Down syndrome to move more efficiently and effectively, feel better about themselves and enjoy their lives more.

Chapter 14
Verbal-motor behaviour in persons with Down syndrome

Brian K.V. Maraj, Shannon D. Robertson, Timothy N. Welsh, Daniel J. Weeks, Romeo Chua, Matthew Heath, Eric A. Roy, Dominic A. Simon, Harold Weinberg and Digby Elliott

Background

Over the last 20 years there have been a number of studies involving children and adults with Down syndrome designed to determine if this unique karyotype influences the pattern of cerebral development and specialization. At least part of this work has been motivated by the notion that atypical patterns of brain organization could be responsible for some of the general, as well as more specific, information processing difficulties experienced by persons from this population. For example, while persons with Down syndrome display many general cognitive problems, they also have particular difficulty (i.e. when compared with other people with intellectual handicaps) performing tasks involving the perception, organization, and production of verbal material (see Elliott, Weeks and Elliott, 1987, for a review).

Because of their specific speech and language difficulties, many of the initial neurobehavioural studies of persons with Down syndrome employed dichotic listening procedures in order to examine cerebral specialization for speech perception. Unlike most persons from the general population, who generally display a right ear/left hemisphere advantage for speech perception, children and adults with Down syndrome were shown to exhibit either left ear/right hemisphere superiority (e.g. Elliott and Weeks, 1993; Hartley, 1981, 1982; Pipe, 1983; Zekulin-Hartley, 1981), or no lateral advantage (e.g. Tannock, Kershner and Oliver, 1984) for the perception of speech sounds. In a 1994 meta-analysis of the dichotic listening studies involving persons with Down syndrome, we found that the reversed pattern of ear advantage was more typical of the 19 experiments completed at that time (Elliott, Weeks and Chua, 1994). Specifically, over this group of studies we found that persons with Down syndrome exhibited a left ear/right hemisphere advantage for speech perception regardless of whether their laterality scores were compared with other handicapped or non-handicapped individuals, or with a theoretical ear difference of zero.

Based on some of the early dichotic listening results, Hartley (1982), and later Pipe (1988) suggested that a reversed pattern of cerebral specialization in persons with Down syndrome may provide the basis for some of the specific speech and language problems exhibited by this group (e.g. Ashman, 1982). The notion was that people with Down syndrome were processing sequential language material with a processing system (i.e. the right cerebral hemisphere) that was not optimal for managing that type of information. Given that it was based exclusively on dichotic listening studies, our research group felt that this model of reversed cerebral specialization was premature. Over the next several years, we examined cerebral specialization in persons with Down syndrome using a number of other noninvasive neuropsychological protocols.

In an initial study (Elliott et al., 1987), we employed a procedure developed by Kinsbourne and Cook (1970; see also Kinsbourne and Hicks, 1978) to investigate cerebral specialization for speech production. We had adult participants perform rapid finger-tapping movements with the right and left index finger in a single-task control condition and while concurrently speaking. Most right-handed people exhibit a slight right hand advantage for finger tapping in the control situation. However, concurrent speech production disrupts right hand, but not left hand performance. This lateralized interference is thought to reflect within-hemisphere interference between left hemisphere systems responsible for the production of speech and those involved in the organization and control of right hand finger movements. Left hand performance is not disrupted by concurrent speech because speech production and control of left hand distal musculature are subserved by different cerebral hemispheres. Given the dichotic listening findings, we were surprised to find this same pattern of interference in adolescents and adults with Down syndrome. Our findings were replicated by Piccirilli et al. (1991) and Parlow, Kinsbourne and Spencer (1996) several years later. Together with the dichotic listening work, these studies indicated that although persons with Down syndrome depend on their right hemisphere for speech perception, their left hemisphere appears to play the executive role in speech production.

Quite recently, we took a different approach to the study of cerebral specialization for speech production in persons with Down syndrome (Heath and Elliott, 1999). This study involved measuring lateral asymmetries in the production of oral movements. Adult participants with and without Down syndrome were videotaped while producing individual (e.g. 'ma'), repeated (e.g. 'ma', 'ma', 'ma' . . .) and sequential (e.g. 'ma', 'ba', 'pi', 'ma', 'ba' . . .) syllables. Kinematic analyses of the videotapes indicated that persons with Down syndrome and control participants exhibited similar mouth asymmetries, with the right side of the mouth opening more quickly and wider than the left side. This asymmetry is thought to reflect left hemisphere innervation of the right side of the face, again indicating left hemisphere specialization for speech production in persons with Down syndrome.

Left hemisphere specialization for speech production is associated with a general lateralized proficiency for specifying the magnitude and timing of muscular force (Elliott and Chua, 1996). It is this superiority in the organization and control of sequential movement that is thought to underlie right-handedness in 90 per cent of the general population (see Elliott and Roy, 1996). Interestingly, while persons with Down syndrome exhibit a slightly higher incidence of left-hand preference than is generally expected (i.e. 15–25 per cent: see Heath, Elliott, Weeks and Chua, 2000, for a review), they generally demonstrate right hand performance advantages similar to persons without Down syndrome of the same chronological age (Elliott, 1985; Elliott, Weeks and Jones, 1986). This finding indicates that for most persons with Down syndrome the left hemisphere plays a special role in the organization and control of both limb and oral movements.

It would appear that persons with Down syndrome perceive speech with their right cerebral hemisphere, but depend on their left cerebral hemisphere for the organization and control of movement. This biological dissociation between speech perception and motor control (including speech production) motivated a series of studies designed to examine any behavioural consequences. In one group of studies, we asked intellectually challenged persons with and without Down syndrome to produce simple limb and oral movements on the basis of either verbal direction or demonstration (Elliott and Weeks, 1990; Elliott, Weeks and Gray, 1990). We videotaped each performance and then used a set of scoring criteria developed by investigators interested in apraxia (Kools, Williams, Vickers and Caell, 1971). The two groups of participants scored equally well when performing the movements based on demonstration, but not when the movements had to be performed following verbal direction. Here the persons with Down syndrome exhibited more movement errors, and this performance difference between the two groups became more pronounced as the number of elements in the movement sequence increased. In a follow-up study, we found that adults with Down syndrome who exhibited the strongest left ear advantage for speech perception exhibited the greatest difficulty with this type of verbal-motor task (Elliott and Weeks, 1993; see also LeClair and Elliott, 1995). Together these findings led us to suggest that verbal-motor impairment associated with Down syndrome results from a breakdown in communication between the cerebral areas responsible for speech perception (right hemisphere) and those responsible for movement organization (left hemisphere). In most of the general population, these two activities are subserved by the same cerebral hemisphere.

Recently our group was fortunate enough to obtain a three-year research grant from the National Down Syndrome Society and the National Institute of Child Health and Human Development to study perceptual-motor behaviour in persons with Down syndrome. Our research programme involves six universities, and specialists in a number of different areas. The grant, as well as the involvement of a number of new investigators, will allow us to test and extend our model of cerebral specialization and perceptual-motor behaviour in persons with Down syndrome. In the remainder of this chapter, we present some of our preliminary findings, as well as some of the future directions of our work.

Verbal-motor behaviour

In a recent study, we attempted to determine if persons with Down syndrome experience problems producing speech on the basis of verbal cues (Bunn et al., submitted). Specifically, we had adults with Down syndrome and control participants of a similar mental and chronological age attempt to speak a series of single syllable words on the basis of written, pictorial and spoken input. The words/pictures were presented at an identical rate in both two- and four-element sets. Either immediately following presentation or after a 5 second retention interval, participants were required to vocally produce the appropriate words in the same order as they were presented (i.e. repeat what they had heard, speak what they had read, or say the word associated with the picture). Each performance was videotaped and scored later for speech errors (e.g. repetitions, pauses, sound prolongations, substitutions, etc.).

Based on our ideas about cerebral organization in persons with Down syndrome, we expected individuals in this group would have greater difficulty than control participants in the repeat condition, because this situation involves both speech perception and speech production. While this result is exactly what we found in the more difficult, four-element sequences, participants with Down syndrome also produced more speech production errors than other participants in the picture condition. Perhaps this finding is associated with the processes involved in attaching a name to the picture (i.e. accessing the lexicon). Further research is currently being conducted to address this unexpected, but interesting finding.

The paradigm most commonly used to investigate the abilities of people to process stimulus information and make a response based on that information is the reaction time paradigm. Typically, the participants in reaction time studies are required to make a movement, either by simply lifting a single finger, or by completing an aiming movement to a target, in response to a particular cue or signal. Although these cues can vary in terms of numbers, complexity, and modality, the key to this paradigm is that the actor must decode the signal, make a decision, and plan, initiate, and complete a response based on that decision. Of interest is the time taken for these processes to be completed, or the total response time. This total response time can be partitioned into two components: reaction time and movement time. Reaction time (RT) is the interval from the stimulus presentation until the response is initiated. Because RT is assumed to reflect the time taken to decode the sensory information, make a decision, and then plan and initiate the response, it is taken as an index of information processing speed within the central nervous system. Movement time, defined as the interval between the initiation and the completion of the movement, depends on the muscular forces involved in the initial impulse and the time taken to use feedback in order to adjust the movement trajectory en route to the target. Thus, movement time usually varies with amplitude of the movement and the size of the target (see Fitts, 1954). However, while traditional assumptions about reaction time and movement time hold that all decision-making processes are completed by the end of the reaction time interval, more recent research has provided evidence to suggest decision-making and response planning can continue into the execution phase of the movement, especially in complex movement situations (e.g. Meegan and Tipper, 1998; Ricker et al., 1999).

In a recent review of the speeded information processing studies involving persons with Down syndrome, Welsh and Elliott (2000) noticed an intriguing pattern of results. Specifically, persons with Down syndrome appear to be slower than other persons of a similar mental age when reacting to auditory but not visual cues or signals. Based on this pattern of results, and our work involving verbal-motor behaviour, a study was designed to examine whether this auditory information processing difficulty extended to situations in which the movement cue was verbal (Welsh and Elliott, in press). A difference between the processing speeds of the verbal information, relative to the visual information, in the persons with Down syndrome would not only be consistent with the previous reaction time findings, but would concur with predictions of verbal-motor difficulties based on the model of biological dissociation (e.g. Chua, Weeks and Elliott, 1996). Specifically, because the areas for speech perception and movement organization are specialized in separate hemispheres, the resulting information transfer between the centres would be slower and less efficient than in those of their peers. For rapid responding based on visual information no difference between the two groups would be expected.

The task involved in this study was to move as quickly as possible to either a blue or a green target. The participants were cued to move to a specific target in three separate ways. The first type of cue was the illumination of the target itself. The second type of cue involved the illumination of either a blue or a green light located next to the origin of the movement. The final type of cue was the auditory presentation of the colour word of the target (e.g. 'blue' or 'green'). The prediction was that the persons with Down syndrome would take longer to respond than their peers with other developmental delays when responding to the verbal movement cues, while no differences were expected to exist when the movement was based on visual information. While we anticipated these modality specific effects to be present in reaction time, the differences between the groups were only found in movement time. Specifically, adults with Down syndrome took longer to acquire the target location than did their normally developing and intellectually impaired counterparts in the verbal, but not in the two visual conditions. This result suggested that, although the sound of the verbal information provided enough alerting information for the participants with Down syndrome to initiate the movement quickly, the full decision–making process (i.e. decoding the speech information and moving to the correct target) was completed while the movement was in progress.

An unexpected finding was that, although there was no difference between the two groups with developmental delays in the condition in which the participants were cued by having the target itself illuminate, the adults with Down syndrome had shorter movement times than their peers when the mapping between visual cue and target was indirect. Again, if differences in movement time are indicative of online decision-making, then adults with Down syndrome appear to be better than their peers with intellectual impairment in using abstract visual information for the programming of movements. This unique finding merits further investigation.

Overall, the results of the Welsh and Elliott (in press) study provide more indirect evidence for the model of biological dissociation (Chua et al., 1996; Elliott, Weeks and Elliott, 1987). In order to examine more specific predictions of the model, we employed a recently developed neuropsychological technique designed to use information processing times to examine information transfer between processing centres within the brain (Welsh, Simon, Watson and Elliott, in preparation). This technique essentially combines the dichotic listening paradigm with the speeded information processing paradigm. For example, in one condition, participants were presented with competing target information to the two ears (i.e. 'blue' presented in one ear and 'green' presented in the other ear). On a particular trial, participants were instructed to pay attention to a specific ear and ignore the information presented to the other ear. As in the previous study, their task was simply to move to the cued green or blue target as rapidly as possible following cue presentation. Based on the assumption that communication between centres within the same hemisphere is faster and more efficient than communication between different hemispheres, persons with Down syndrome were expected to exhibit a different pattern of response times than other participants.

Adults without Down syndrome were expected to perform the movement task more quickly and exhibit the fewest errors when responding with their right hand to targets presented to the right ear, because in this group the left cerebral hemisphere subserves both speech perception and the organization and control of right hand movements. Consistent with previous dichotic research, we anticipated that persons with Down syndrome would demonstrate a left ear, and perhaps left hand, advantage for reaction time, movement time and movement errors. However, the results of the study were not as predicted. Specifically, we found that the persons with and without Down syndrome demonstrated superior performance when attending to the right ear.

Because this finding of a right ear advantage in persons with Down syndrome was unusual, we had the same participants complete a more traditional, free recall dichotic listening task. This test was performed post hoc in order to investigate whether responsibility for the anomalous finding rested on the participants or on the task (cf. Elliott et al., 1994). The results of this test revealed, as had been previously shown, that the persons with Down syndrome had an overall left ear advantage for the perception of speech sounds. Surprisingly, there was a robust positive correlation between the laterality indices generated for the two tasks. Thus, while the relative position of individual scores was maintained, ear advantages for the dichotic movement task were shifted towards left hemisphere dominance.

Upon a closer examination of the results for the dichotic movement task, an interesting pattern emerged. Although the adults with Down syndrome did have shorter reaction times and fewer movement errors when concentrating on the right ear, they also performed better in situations in which intrahemispheric communication could be used to complete the task. That is, persons with Down syndrome performed better in the right ear/right hand condition than in the right ear/left hand condition, and better in the left ear/left hand condition than in the left ear/right hand condition. Thus, while one hemisphere may be dominant for the performance of each task separately, it appears that each hemisphere has the ability to complete both the speech perception and movement organization components of the overall task. In this situation at least, within-hemisphere task completion appears to have its advantages (see Jones and Elliott, 1988). In the case of persons with Down syndrome, this type of within-hemisphere processing may reflect an adaptive strategy (see Latash and Anson, 1996) adopted by the central nervous system to deal with interhemispheric communication difficulties related to a smaller corpus callosum (Wang, Doherty, Hesselink and Bellugi, 1992). Once again, this hypothesis provides a direction for our future research.

Motor learning

In the majority of our work on verbal-motor behaviour in persons with Down syndrome, we have concentrated our efforts on studying motor performance, or how an individual is able to perform a movement task at one point in time. Of greater practical relevance is how various sources of information contribute to motor learning: that is, to stable changes in performance following practice. In motor learning research concerned with feedback in the form of knowledge of results (e.g. Salmoni, Schmidt and Walter, 1984), and practice structure (e.g. Lee and Magill, 1983), it has been demonstrated that conditions that facilitate motor performance are not always optimal for long-term retention of a motor skill or transfer of learning to a similar movement task. One goal of our research programme has thus been to determine if the specific problems that persons with Down syndrome have with verbal-motor performance generalize to verbal-motor learning.

In an initial learning study, we taught adults with and without Down syndrome a novel three-element movement sequence using a verbal instructional protocol (Elliott, Gray and Weeks, 1991). The goal was to complete the task as quickly as possible. During the acquisition phase of the study participants were cued verbally about the movement to be completed prior to each attempt and they were given verbal feedback about their performance. Following 45 practice trials (five blocks of nine trials) and a short rest interval, we examined retention of the newly learned skill in a situation in which verbal cueing and feedback were no longer available. These retention conditions were designed to approximate what would happen in a real learning situation when the instructor is no longer present to guide the learner through each performance. As in the aiming studies discussed earlier, we measured the time to initiate the movement sequence (reaction time) and the time to execute the movement sequence (movement time), as well as the number of movement sequencing errors. Our retention results revealed that while persons with Down syndrome executed their movements just as quickly and accurately as control participants of a similar mental and chronological age, they took longer to initiate each movement sequence.[1] This finding was our first indication that some of the difficulties persons with Down syndrome have organizing movements on the basis of verbal direction (e.g. LeClair and Elliott, 1995) also influence their ability to learn a novel motor task.

One of the shortcomings of our 1991 study was that while it was concerned with verbal-motor learning, it did not include a control learning situation in which instruction was provided in another manner. In a very recent experiment, we addressed that problem by using both a verbal and visual instructional protocol (Maraj, Li, Hillman and Johnson, under review). The task was a computer-based movement sequence in which the participants had to move the cursor (via a mouse) to three targets that were arranged vertically on the computer screen. Child and adult participants of a similar mental age were instructed to move to the targets from the home position. On each trial, the sequence was prompted either verbally (e.g. 'middle', 'top', 'bottom') or participants were shown a visual demonstration (the program was designed to move the cursor automatically to the required locations). The learner had to reproduce the sequence they were shown or told as quickly and accurately as possible after the sound of a tone.

In the acquisition phase of the study, participants with Down syndrome were slower at initiating their movements in the verbal condition as compared with participants of a similar mental age with undifferentiated mental disabilities and those who were non-handicapped. Persons with Down syndrome performed better in the visual situation than when the movement cues were provided verbally. Participants in both intellectually handicapped groups were slower to move than persons in the non-handicapped group. These performance results are consistent with other verbal-motor findings as well as with our model of cerebral organization for persons with Down syndrome. Contrary to our previous work, however (e.g. Elliott et al., 1991), persons with Down syndrome were no slower than persons of a similar mental and chronological age at initiating their movements during retention at 1 hour and 24 hours regardless of how they had been trained (i.e. visually or verbally). Thus, at least in terms of reaction time, the verbal-motor performance problem did not generalize to motor learning. Moreover, persons with Down syndrome were able to initiate their movements just as rapidly as their peers of a similar mental and chronological age when they

---

[1] The apparent inconsistency between the reaction time and movement time in this learning study as compared with Welsh and Elliott (in press) may relate to the fact that the sequencing task was always the same and thus required no decision-making. In the Welsh and Elliott study, participants may have been leaving the home position before deciding on the target.

were required to perform movement sequences during transfer conditions. In this study, transfer involved performing the movement sequence following cueing via the untrained modality (i.e. verbal cueing of the visually trained participants and vice versa). Regardless of the learning, retention, or transfer condition, control participants without intellectual handicaps initiated their movements more quickly than persons in the two handicapped groups.

The movement time findings during acquisition were very similar to the reaction time results. That is, persons with Down syndrome took longer to complete their movements in the verbal condition than in the visual condition, but were slightly better than their peers of a similar mental age in the former situation. Both groups were slower than participants without mental handicaps.

Perhaps the most interesting results are evident in movement times during retention and transfer. In the retention test, participants were tested at 1 hour and 24 hours after the acquisition trials in the same condition (visual/verbal) in which they practised the movement sequence. The results showed that participants with Down syndrome were slower in the verbal condition as compared with the visual condition. Persons with Down syndrome did not differ from participants in the other handicapped group in the verbal condition at 1 hour, but at 24 hours, unlike other participants, persons with Down syndrome showed a tremendous increase in movement time. There were no group differences under visual conditions. These findings suggest that as time went along, the learning derived from conditions of verbal instruction experienced greater decay in the people with Down syndrome. In fact, time seemed to exacerbate an already challenging mode of information presentation for persons with Down syndrome.

In the transfer test, participants were also tested at 1 hour and 24 hours after the acquisition trials. However, the participants who had acquisition trials in the verbal condition were switched to the visual condition and those in the visual condition were switched to the verbal condition. The results indicated that the visual instruction resulted in superior learning. Participants who had practised with vision transferred easily to the verbal condition. They also demonstrated superior performance to the participants who practised in the verbal situation and switched to the visual condition. The effect was even more pronounced after 24 hours. The group that practised in the visual condition was able to easily transfer to the verbal condition after 1 day with no decay. In fact, their performance was significantly better after 24 hours than after 1 hour.

We interpret this robust effect of the visual condition in transfer as consistent with our model of cerebral organization in persons with Down syndrome. While prompted modality appears to be important, we need to further investigate if long-term effects in transfer across learning mode can be

seen in other variations of movement task dimensions. Our future work will
continue to explore the means by which long-term retention and transfer can
be facilitated in the acquisition of movement skill for functionally relevant
activities for persons with Down syndrome.

Coordinating limb movements

It has been suggested that because of the dissociation of auditory/speech
perception and movement production, individuals with Down syndrome
may perform movement skills more accurately when prompted with visual as
opposed to auditory/speech information (Elliott and Weeks, 1993; Elliott et
al., 1994). To date, however, most of our research has focused on discrete,
unimanual tasks (Elliott, 1985; Elliott and Weeks, 1990). One goal of our
current research is to determine whether or not our findings involving
discrete tasks extend to more continuous movements that involve the coordination of the limbs with each other or with an external event.

In an initial coordination study, we examined how persons with and
without Down syndrome were able to coordinate an arm movement with a
visual and an auditory metronome (Chua et al., 1996). One purpose of this
study was to determine whether purely auditory information, as opposed to
verbal information, caused perceptual-motor difficulties in individuals with
Down syndrome (see Welsh and Elliott, 2000). The task was to perform
rhythmic left to right movements with the forearm using a lever. The participants were instructed to synchronize their movement with the metronome.
The visual metronome consisted of a cursor that flashed, alternating between
the left and right side of a computer monitor. The auditory metronome was a
1000 Hz tone that sounded with the same cycling frequency as the visual
metronome (once every second). Each trial began with both the visual and
auditory metronome present. After 15 cycles (2 seconds each), either the
visual or auditory metronome continued alone for another 15 cycles. A
measure of coordination (relative phase) between the hand movements and
the metronome was calculated. The results suggested that, contrary to the
model's predictions, some participants actually exhibited better coordination
with the auditory metronome. These pilot data indicated that adults with
Down syndrome do not have specific problems in coordinating movements
to an auditory metronome.

Recently we have conducted a follow-up study (Robertson et al., under
review) involving bimanual coordination. In this study, young adults and
adolescents with Down syndrome and groups of control participants of a
similar mental age and a similar chronological age performed a bimanual
circle drawing task. This movement task was paced by either an auditory or a
visual metronome. The participants' task was to draw one circle every time a

beep sounded (auditory metronome) or a circle flashed (visual metronome). During a trial, the metronomes were initially paced at 1000 ms intervals for 10 seconds, then increased to 800 ms for 10 seconds and finally increased to 600 ms for 10 seconds. The time to complete one circle revealed that participants of a similar chronological age without intellectual impairment increased their speed according to the metronome. However, the persons with Down syndrome and their counterparts of a similar mental age performed at a speed that they were comfortable with and maintained that speed throughout the trial. A spatial measure indicating the circularity of the circle was also calculated (Franz, Zelaznik and McCabe, 1991). For this measure, there were differences between the two metronome conditions. The participants in both control groups produced shapes that were more circular with the visual metronome, whereas persons with Down syndrome drew shapes that were more circular with the auditory metronome. A measure of coordination between the hands (relative phase), which takes into account temporal and spatial aspects of the task, revealed a similar effect of the metronomes. The control participants were more accurate in coordinating their two hands with the visual metronome, whereas persons with Down syndrome were more accurate coordinating their hands with the auditory metronome.

These results are quite different from those involving discrete auditory-motor tasks (see Welsh and Elliott, 2000, for a review), and suggest that auditory-motor problems associated with Down syndrome may be limited to discrete motor tasks and/or are peculiar to auditory tasks that involve verbal decoding (LeClair and Elliott, 1995; Welsh and Elliott, 2000). However, another interpretation of these results is possible when one considers that persons with Down syndrome did better with the auditory metronome only with respect to the spatial components of the task. If vision is assumed to be critical for producing circular movements, it could be the case that the visual metronome actually interfered with performance by drawing visual attention away from the movements the two arms were required to complete (see Hodges et al., 1995, and Kulatunga-Moruzi and Elliott, 1999). Recall that, in terms of timing, the performance of persons with Down syndrome was independent of metronome speed anyway. Thus, better spatial performance with the auditory metronome for persons with Down syndrome could be because auditory information is simply less salient, in this case less distracting. This interpretation of the results is consistent with models proposing that attention has a limited capacity (Kahneman, 1973; Wickens, 1984) and plays a major role in the performance of motor skills. Also, there is a body of research indicating that individuals with developmental handicaps are not able to focus their attention as well as other people of a similar mental age (Merrill and O'Dekirk, 1994). In future research we plan to investigate the influence of visual information and attention on spatial and non-spatial continuous tasks in individuals with Down syndrome.

Electrophysiological assessment of cerebral specialization

To date we have attempted to remain mindful of maintaining at least a minimum of neurophysiological relevance in developing our neuropsychological model of biological dissociation (Elliott, Weeks and Elliott, 1987). However, fully realizing the theoretical and clinical implications of our behavioural work on information processing in individuals with Down syndrome (cf. Chua, Weeks and Elliott, 1996) demands that we explore such relevance in greater detail. To that end, we are beginning to investigate the locus and nature of the brain–behaviour relations originally established through the behavioural, neuropsychological research. By examining the electrical activity of the brain, the goal is to associate a description of information processing events with a description of brain function.

Recent advances in brain-imaging techniques have provided investigators with effective tools for identification and localization of active neural systems in the brain during the performance of certain cognitive and motor tasks. Advances in electroencephalography (EEG), as well as the rapid development of biomagnetic technology such as magnetoencephalography (MEG), provide non-invasive methods with which to examine cerebral activity. The EEG and MEG, with their high temporal resolution, are particularly suited for the examination of time-evolving dynamics of cortical activity. The MEG, which measures transient changes in the magnetic flux generated by intracellular electrical currents in large neuronal aggregates, further enhances the spatial resolution afforded by EEG. Variations in the strength of scalp-recorded magnetic flux are recorded as event-related magnetic fields and progress in analytical methods such as source (dipole) localization has also enhanced our window into the neural systems' underlying behaviour.

Recently, we conducted a review of structural and functional neuroimaging research (Gaetz et al., under review) as a first step in substantiating the behavioural anomalies associated with Down syndrome. Because of the importance that our model of biological dissociation places on the relative costs and benefits associated with visual versus verbal modes of instruction in the performance of perceptual-motor tasks, we are particularly interested in the processing of linguistic material by persons with Down syndrome. One striking aspect of the available literature is the consistency among studies of brain structure and function, in addition to behavioural data, suggesting that functional language deficits in persons with Down syndrome stem from specific decrements in traditional language structures.

More specifically, the triplication of at least the distal portion of the long arm of chromosome 21 apparently leads to abnormal dendritic spine morphology as well as irregular migration of inhibitory cells in various cortical areas including those involved in language. One scenario is that abnormalities in migration and development of excitatory and inhibitory cells occurring at a critical developmental period may lead to disrupted organization of both local circuits and neural systems connections which, in turn, contributes to specific language deficits (Gaetz et al., under review).

Such aberrant migration of inhibitory cells is also consistent with most electrophysiological studies of persons with Down syndrome. What emerges from several studies is that, regardless of sensory modality, there is a pattern of reduced latency of early evoked potentials, increased latency of later peaks, larger peak amplitudes in averaged and single trials, and little habituation of responses. The latter is particularly interesting in that it is consistent with the disruption of inhibitory cells that occurs with Down syndrome. Taken together, the available evidence suggests that differences in central inhibition of afferent stimuli characterize the brain in persons with Down syndrome. Lack of habituation to repetitive stimulation is indicative of reduced inhibitory control, reduced selectivity and specificity of responsiveness, slower processing, abnormal temporal integration as well as storage and integration of certain types of information. When the evidence is integrated, there is reason to believe that the deficit may primarily be associated with systems involved in the processing of language and speech sounds. This suggestion is consistent with behavioural work from several laboratories, including our own, which shows a greater right hemisphere involvement in language perception in persons with Down syndrome. Indeed, this feature is central to our model of biological dissociation. Moreover, this notion is consistent with positron-emission tomography (PET) data that demonstrate abnormal left hemisphere function and greater right hemisphere involvement during language processing (e.g. Horwitz, Schapiro, Grady and Rapoport, 1990). In addition, studies involving EEG frequency analysis show a consistent deficit in alpha activity with more power in other frequencies compared with control subjects without Down syndrome. New findings suggest that understanding alpha activity may have important implications for understanding speech perception since there may be a special role for alpha responses in primary sensory processing (e.g. Bashar et al., 1999).

In a recent empirical effort from our laboratory (Weinberg et al., under review), MEG was used to image brain function during the performance of a receptive language task and while listening to 'clicks' that were presented in the right ear, the left ear, or in both ears. For the language task real and nonsense words were randomly presented. Concatenating the real words resulted in a coherent story. Images of the distribution of magnetic fields were constructed for selected time intervals during the processing of language stimuli and for specific components of the response to auditory stimuli. Equivalent dipole estimates were computed for each of the distributions and plotted in a sphere that approximated the brain, thus localizing the sources of the distributions in the space of the brain.

Responses to bilateral auditory stimulation (the clicks) showed abnormal topography when compared with individuals without Down syndrome. Further, significant time delay in arrival of sensory information to cortical areas is observed during right ear stimulation, suggesting abnormal subcortical processing in Down syndrome. The equivalent current sources associated with auditory processing were displaced anteriorly when compared with individuals without Down syndrome. Most interesting was the response to language processing, which revealed a right hemisphere bias. In another study currently underway we have gathered both EEG and MEG data (Weeks et al., in preparation) using the procedure of Bunn et al. (submitted) described earlier in this chapter. In separate blocks of trials, adult participants with and without Down syndrome were required to verbally announce the stimulus that had been presented to them in picture, text or spoken form. Image maps of cortical activity were generated in a sphere that approximated the brain. While considerably more analyses are required to determine the effect of the different modes of presentation, when compared with persons without Down syndrome, the participants with Down syndrome showed consistent and dramatic reversals of current flow between the stimulus presentation and response preparation intervals for all presentation modes. These shifts represent changes in inter- and intra-hemispheric interactions during completion of the task that are not observed in the control participants.

In summary, although we prefer to remain cautious in our conclusions, the suggestion is that the organization of active systems required for performance in these language/speech tasks is indeed qualitatively different in Down syndrome compared with what would be expected in normal individuals and is not inconsistent with the tenets of our behavioural model of cerebral specialization (Elliott, Weeks and Elliott, 1987). As further analyses of these data begin to influence the development and theoretical direction of our model it may be that, rather than thinking about isolated centres of processing, the implications of the dissociation model may be better realized by an analysis of the dynamic information flow and frequency spectra of the magnetic fields associated with task performance.

Summary and conclusions

During the late 1980s and early 1990s, we slowly developed a picture of how verbal-motor processing in persons with Down syndrome differs from other individuals of a similar mental and chronological age. Our work led us to propose a simple model of cerebral function in persons with Down syndrome that we have used to guide our neurobehavioural research, including much of the research presented in this chapter. With the recent support of the National Down Syndrome Society and the National Institute of Child Health and Human Development, our programme of research has grown dramatically in the last two years. Empirical, theoretical and technical contributions now come from a team of investigators representing six major universities, with a much broader range of expertise. While many of our new findings are consistent with our early ideas about perceptual-motor behaviour in persons with Down syndrome, it is also clear that our model of cerebral organization is too simple to explain many of our most recent behavioural and neuroimaging findings described here. We are currently in the midst of a number of empirical investigations designed to resolve the outstanding issues raised in the various sections of this chapter. It is to be hoped that these experiments will provide the basis for a more encompassing theoretical contribution on verbal-motor behaviour in persons with Down syndrome, perhaps before the next World Congress.

References

Ashman AF (1982) Coding, strategic behavior and language performance of institutionalized mentally retarded young adults. American Journal of Mental Deficiency 86: 627-36.

Bashar E, Demiral T, Schuermann M, Basar-Eroglu C, Ademoglu A (1999) Oscillatory brain dynamics, wavelet analysis, and cognition. Brain and Language 66: 146-83.

Bunn L, Welsh TN, Watson C, Simon DA, Elliott D (submitted for publication) Speech production errors in adults with and without Down syndrome following verbal, written, and pictorial cues. Available from T Welsh.

Chua R, Weeks DJ, Elliott D (1996) A functional systems approach to understanding verbal-motor integration in individuals with Down syndrome. Down Syndrome: Research and Practice 4: 25-36.

Elliott D (1985) Manual asymmetries in the performance of sequential movements by adolescents and adults with Down syndrome. American Journal of Mental Deficiency 90: 90-7.

Elliott D, Chua R (1996) Manual asymmetries in goal-directed movement. In Elliott D, Roy EA (Eds) Manual Asymmetries in Motor Performance. Boca Raton: CRC Press. pp 143-58.

Elliott D, Edwards JM, Weeks DJ, Lindley S, Carnahan H (1987) Cerebral specialization in young adults with Down syndrome. American Journal on Mental Retardation 91: 480-5.

Elliott D, Gray S, Weeks DJ (1991) Verbal cueing and motor skill acquisition for adults with Down syndrome. Adapted Physical Activity Quarterly 8: 210-20.

Elliott D, Roy EA (1996) Manual Asymmetries in Motor Performance. Boca Raton: CRC Press.

Elliott D, Weeks DJ (1990) Cerebral specialization and the control of oral and limb movements for individuals with Down's syndrome. Journal of Motor Behavior 22: 6-18.

Elliott D, Weeks DJ (1993) Cerebral specialization for speech perception and movement organization in adults with Down's syndrome. Cortex 29: 103-13.

Elliott D, Weeks DJ, Chua R (1994) Anomalous cerebral lateralization and Down syndrome. Brain and Cognition 26: 191-5.

Elliott D, Weeks DJ, Elliott CL (1987) Cerebral specialization in young adults with Down syndrome. American Journal on Mental Retardation 92: 263-71.

Elliott D, Weeks DJ, Gray S (1990) Manual and oral praxis in adults with Down's syndrome. Neuropsychologia 28: 1307-15.

Elliott D, Weeks DJ, Jones R (1986) Lateral asymmetries in finger-tapping by adolescents and young adults with Down syndrome. American Journal of Mental Deficiency 90: 472-5.

Fitts PM (1954) The information capacity of the human motor system in controlling the amplitude of movement. Journal of Experimental Psychology 47: 381-91.

Franz EA, Zelaznik HN, McCabe G (1991) Spatial topological constraints in a bimanual task. Acta Psychologica 77: 137-51.

Gaetz M, Weeks DJ, Chua R, Weinberg H, Welsh T, Elliott D (under review) Structural and functional evidence for language dysfunction in Down syndrome: a review of neuroimaging research. Available from D Weeks.

Hartley XY (1981) Lateralization of speech stimuli in young Down's syndrome children. Cortex 17: 241-8.

Hartley XY (1982) Receptive language processing of Down's syndrome children. Journal of Mental Deficiency Research 26: 263-9.

Heath M, Elliott D (1999) Cerebral specialization for speech production in persons with Down syndrome. Brain and Language 69: 193-211.

Heath M, Elliott D, Weeks DJ, Chua R (2000) A functional systems approach to movement pathology in persons with Down syndrome. In Weeks DJ, Chua R, Elliott D (Eds) Perceptual-motor Behavior in Down Syndrome. Champaign, IL: Human Kinetics. pp 305-20.

Hodges NJ, Cunningham SJ, Lyons J, Kerr TL, Elliott D (1995) Visual feedback processing and goal-directed movement in adults with Down syndrome. Adapted Physical Activity Quarterly 12: 176-86.

Horwitz B, Schapiro MB, Grady CL, Rapoport SI (1990) Cerebral metabolic pattern in young adult Down's syndrome subjects: altered intercorrelations between regional rates of glucose utilization. Journal on Mental Deficiency Research 34: 237-52.

Jones R, Elliott D (1988) Intra- and inter-hemispheric integration of tactual and visual spatial information. Bulletin of the Psychonomic Society 26: 229-31.

Kahneman D (1973) Attention and Effort. Englewood Cliffs, NJ: Prentice Hall.

Kinsbourne M, Cook J (1970) Generalized and lateralized effects of concurrent cognitive activity on a unimanual skill. Cortex 11: 283-90.

Kinsbourne M, Hicks RE (1978) Functional cerebral space: a model for overflow, transfer and interference effects in human performance. In Requin J (Ed) Attention and Performance, VII. New York: Academic Press. pp 345-62.

Kools JA, Williams AF, Vickers MJ, Caell A (1971) Oral and limb apraxia in mentally retarded children with deviant articulation. Cortex 7: 387–400.

Kulatunga-Moruzi C, Elliott D (1999) Manual and attentional asymmetries in goal-directed movements in adults with Down syndrome. Adapted Physical Activity Quarterly 16: 138–54.

Latash ML, Anson JG (1996) What are 'normal movements' in atypical populations? Behavioral and Brain Sciences 19: 55–106.

LeClair DA, Elliott D (1995) Movement preparation and the costs and benefits associated with advance information for adults with Down syndrome. Adapted Physical Activity Quarterly 12: 238–49.

Lee TD, Magill RA (1983) The locus of contextual interference in motor skill acquisition. Journal of Experimental Psychology: Learning, Memory and Cognition 9: 730–46.

Maraj BKV, Li L, Hillman R, Johnson J (under review). Visual and verbal instruction in the acquisition of a sequential movement task. Available from B Maraj.

Meegan DV, Tipper SP (1998) Reaching in cluttered visual environments: spatial and temporal influences of distracting objects. Quarterly Journal of Experimental Psychology: Human Experimental Psychology 51A: 225–49.

Merrill EC, O'Dekirk JM (1994) Visual selective attention and mental retardation. Cognitive Neuropsychology 11: 117–32.

Parlow SE, Kinsbourne M, Spencer J (1996) Cerebral laterality in adults with severe mental retardation. Developmental Neuropsychology 12: 299–312.

Piccirilli M, D'Alessandro P, Mazzi P, Sciarma T, Testa A (1991) Cerebral organization for language in Down's syndrome patients. Cortex 27: 41–7.

Pipe ME (1983) Dichotic-listening performance following auditory discrimination training in Down's syndrome and developmentally retarded children. Cortex 19: 481–91.

Pipe ME (1988) Atypical laterality and retardation. Psychological Bulletin 104: 343–9.

Ricker KL, Elliott D, Lyons J, Gauldie D, Chua R, Byblow W (1999) The utilization of visual information in the control of rapid sequential aiming movements. Acta Psychologica 103: 103–23.

Robertson SD, Winges JB, Kao JC, Weeks DJ, Chua R (under review) Asymmetrical cerebral organization in individuals with Down syndrome: application to continuous and bimanual tasks. Available from S Robertson.

Salmoni AW, Schmidt RA, Walter CB (1984) Knowledge of results and motor learning: a review and critical appraisal. Psychological Bulletin 95: 355–86.

Tannock R, Kershner JR, Oliver J (1984) Do individuals with Down's syndrome possess right hemisphere language dominance? Cortex 20: 221–31.

Wang PP, Doherty S, Hesselink JR, Bellugi U (1992) Callosal morphology concurs with neurobehavioral and neuropsychological findings in two neurodevelopmental disorders. Archives of Neurology 49: 407–11.

Weeks DJ, Chua R, Weinberg H, Cheyne D, Welsh T, Schneider T, Sturrock S, Elliott D (in preparation) EEG and MEG assessment of cerebral specialisation for receptive and expressive language in individuals with Down syndrome. Available from D Weeks.

Weinberg H, Weeks DJ, Chua R, Cheyne D, Elliott D (under review) The use of magnetoencephalography (MEG) to investigate cerebral specialization in Down syndrome. Available from H Weinberg.

Welsh TN, Elliott D (2000) The preparation and control of goal-directed limb movements in persons with Down syndrome. In Weeks DJ, Chua R, Elliott D (Eds) Perceptual-motor Behavior in Down Syndrome. Champaign, IL: Human Kinetics. pp 49–70.

Welsh TN, Elliott D (in press) The processing speed of visual and verbal movement stimuli by adults with and without Down syndrome. Adapted Physical Activity Quarterly.

Welsh TN, Simon D, Watson C, Elliott D (in preparation) Cerebral specialization and verbal-motor integration in adults with and without Down syndrome. Available from T Welsh.

Wickens CD (1984) Processing resources in attention. In Parasuraman R, Davies DR (Eds) Varieties of Attention. New York: Academic Press. pp 63–102.

Zekulin-Hartley XY (1981) Hemispheric asymmetry in Down's syndrome children. Canadian Journal of Behavioural Science 13: 210–17.

SECTION 8
SERVICE DEVELOPMENT

Introduction

Roy McConkey reminds us that although things have changed remarkably for individuals with Down syndrome in the western world these same changes have not occurred for those in developing countries. He points out that the lives of people with a disability are not a priority for governments in these countries as other needs are seen to be more pressing. Nevertheless, he suggests that there are ways forward available to individual services working for people with a disability in these countries. McConkey argues that we must recognize and then use the strengths of the communities in which they live to better the lives of individuals with a disability. The goals for intervention must reflect the goals of the society in which the individual lives, and the mechanisms for intervention must also spring from within the community.

McConkey enumerates the particular challenges that make it difficult for communities in developing countries to develop effective services. He also identifies traditional strengths within developing countries that can be harnessed for the benefit of individuals with a disability and their families. He then proposes three strategies that he argues should be used to alter the circumstances of those with a disability: family involvement, mobilizing communities, and the development of national policies that take the needs of individuals with a disability into consideration. In his practical way, McConkey explains a number of methods that might be used to operationalize these strategies, generally drawing on the strengths he had earlier identified. Finally, he urges that the efforts of those working in developing countries be concentrated on the three 'E's - early intervention, education and employment.

CHAPTER 15
Creating positive lifestyles for people with Down syndrome in developing countries

ROY MCCONKEY

Down syndrome occurs in every society of the world and has done so for centuries. In years gone by, many babies born with the syndrome died soon after birth as they succumbed to various diseases: a risk that still prevails in many poorer countries to this day. Of course many were not recognized as having Down syndrome, but their obvious impairments marked them out as being different from other babies. They shared the same fate of other impaired youngsters: often hidden away because of the shame a defective child brought to the family. These children were thus dually disadvantaged, initially by their impairment and then subsequently by the lack of learning opportunities.

Today the picture is changing, albeit more rapidly in some countries than in others. This chapter focuses on less affluent nations sometimes referred to as the third world, non-industrialized societies or developing countries. However, there is a sense in which all the world's nations are still developing in their response to people with disabilities in general and those with Down syndrome in particular. Indeed, until 30 years ago the opening paragraph was just as applicable to the rich counties.

This chapter reviews the critical strategies that are transforming the future of people with Down syndrome from one of despair and hopelessness to a valued and positive lifestyle in their family and the community.

Challenges facing developing countries

Before discussing how this goal may be met, we do need to acknowledge that developing nations face some particular challenges in responding to the needs of people with Down syndrome. These challenges, listed below, impact at every level of service provision and need to be addressed directly when changes intended to lead to improvements in the lives of those with Down syndrome are considered.

Lack of resources

The health, education and social services of many countries struggle to cope with their citizens' ordinary needs let alone the more intricate and individual requirements of those with disabilities. Hence 'low tech' solutions will continue to be needed for the foreseeable future (Werner, 1987).

Lack of expertise

The affluent world is rich in professional expertise, a heritage handed down from previous generations who developed training opportunities and career structures that are emulated by a growing number of specialisms. But this is not the case for poorer nations. Rather, disability services are dependent on whatever personnel are available locally, sometimes with support from overseas workers funded by international agencies on short-term contracts. It is humbling for overseas visitors to realize that so much has been – and can be – achieved with relatively few resources. In my experience, the best value-for-money services are those in developing countries simply because they can't afford to waste a cent!

Lack of priority

Given the many demands on all governments for better health, education for all, and full employment, it is no surprise that people with disabilities are a low priority for increased state funding. However, reliance on fund-raising at home or abroad sustains the notion of helplessness that features in many donors' images of disability (Brohier, 1995), and therefore should be avoided where possible.

Coleridge (1993) recommended two strategies for making disability more of a priority issue. First, disability advocates and associations need to come together in alliances to press their case. Second, disability concerns should feature in *all* community development initiatives, for example, education, housing or employment, rather than trying to argue for a unique response for those with a particular disability. Sad to say, neither of these two strategies is much used in affluent countries. There disability groups are more inclined to defend their own corner and promote their particular concerns than to find common cause with like-minded allies. Perhaps the developing world can show that cooperation is preferable to competition.

Strengths of developing countries

The foregoing analysis would be incomplete without assessing the strengths that are inherent in many developing countries and which make them rich in comparison with the so-called developed world.

Supportive families

The culture of supportive families remains strong in many places throughout the developing world. Extended families are available to assist with practical aspects of life such as child-minding as well as offering the emotional and social support that is needed by first-time parents. The family also provides a measure of economic security, as self-sufficiency is essential for survival in most countries.

Community structures

The sense of belonging to a community also remains strong in most developing countries, nurtured as it is through force of economic inter-dependency but also by religious faith, community celebrations and festivals. Moreover, health services and schools serve the local community; rarely is there the option to use services in other locations, as transport is not readily available.

Freedom from precedent

Many developing countries have little or no history of responding to disability. This is unlike the developed world where much energy and effort has to be expended on dismantling old ways of helping people with disabilities – institutional care is probably the best example. Rather, creative ways of meeting people's needs can be attempted and local solutions found.

Of course, these generalizations do not apply in all countries, or even in all parts of a country, but even if they are not immediately apparent, the challenge for anyone involved in helping people with disability is to try to generate these three strengths. This is very much the thrust of policy in many affluent countries as they shift from institutional to community-based care (Schwartz, 1992). Ironically, the poorer nations of the world may stand a better chance of bringing such policies to fruition because of their wealth in family and community.

Three strategies are recommended in this paper for building on the identified strengths of developing countries, therefore making the priorities for intervention more realizable. These are family involvement; the mobilizing of communities; and the institution of national policies to promote the rights of people with disabilities. As you will discover, these apply as much to the developed as to the developing world.

Strategy 1: Family involvement

All families, no matter how poor or impoverished are involved when a child has Down syndrome. Perhaps the mistake that was made in the past was thinking that specialists rather than family members were needed to cope with the child's special needs arising from the impairments associated with Down syndrome. We know that the involvement of specialists does make a difference, but when they attempt to intervene without involving families in promoting the child's development the outcomes are much less effective (Gallagher, 1990). Hence the first strategy for creating positive lifestyles is to involve families in promoting the child's development and well-being. Of course when specialist help is non-existent, there is no alternative but to rely on families.

The rationale for involving families is simply stated.

- They are the primary supporters of the person with Down syndrome now and probably throughout their lifetime.
- Their attitudes and beliefs will profoundly affect the lifestyle and opportunities open to the person with disabilities in their community – for better or for worse.
- Research has shown that nearly all families have the competence and potential to nurture the physical, social, emotional and intellectual well-being of children with disabilities just as they do with typically developing children. White (1979) for example, summarized the outcome of his research in promoting the development of 'at risk' preschoolers in the United States when he wrote:

> We came to believe that the informal education which parents provide for their children makes more of an impact on the child's total educational development than does the formal education system.

How can families become more effective in promoting their child's development? In recent years, experience and research from around the world has demonstrated the value of two types of help especially during the childhood years: the use of home visitors, and the formation of parent associations.

Although these are considered separately in this paper, they are not meant to be alternatives but rather they should form a coherent response to family needs from as early in the child's life as possible.

Home visitors

One of the most powerful ways of involving families is through the use of what is often called 'home visitors'. Their role is to advise and guide the family on coping with the disability. This may mean informing families about the help that is available in the locality, such as hospital clinics. They may recommend equipment or aids to assist the person, such as a walking frame, or demonstrate exercises or learning activities that the family can use at home to help the person acquire new skills.

By visiting the family regularly, for example every two weeks, the home visitor can build a trusting relationship with the carers – usually the child's mother or grandmother. The role may then extend into one of counselling mothers, listening to their concerns and advising on marital difficulties, financial problems and hurtful reactions of family members or neighbours.

Home visitors are not a new concept, of course. The extended family or 'tribe' has often provided an adviser or confidante to new mothers with whom they can discuss their concerns. The home visiting concept builds on this tradition by introducing the family to a person who has particular expertise or interest in their child's condition. However, societies vary in their tolerance of an 'outsider' becoming involved in family issues and services must be sensitive to this when recruiting staff to act as home visitors (Jaffer and Jaffer, 1990).

Equally, the role can be demanding, and the effectiveness of the home visitor will depend not only on their personal qualities but also on the training they receive, a topic to which I return below. (See Thorburn, 1990, for a discussion of the role of home visitors.)

Home visitors can be recruited from at least three different sources, and projects around the world invariably use some combination of the ones outlined here.

Existing personnel

Re-deploying existing personnel to act as home visitors has been a popular option in affluent countries. Teachers, therapists and health workers have adopted this new style of working. The strategy has been successful also in developing countries. In one of the islands of the Philippines, teachers who previously worked in a special school were retrained as home visitors and allocated to various districts where they visited the children at home or in ordinary schools to support the parents and teachers in their work.

Paid staff

Many community projects have devoted resources to the recruitment, training and employment of individuals to act as home visitors to families and people with disabilities. This is the concept underpinning the World Health Organization model of Community Based Rehabilitation (Helander, 1993). Although the original idea was to recruit people from the community, in later years an increasing number of people with disabilities or parents of children with disabilities have successfully been employed as home visitors (McGlade and Acquino, 1995). This strategy not only gives much needed employment opportunities but these individuals come with personal insights and motivation which can make them more effective and also more acceptable to families.

Volunteer workers

The use of volunteer workers forms a third option. Once again, some community services use family members as their primary workers, an idea that is also prevalent in more affluent countries where parents work alongside professionals when families first learn that their child has a disability. However, other community schemes have successfully recruited teachers and health workers, among others, to act as supporters for families. This is best exemplified in O'Toole's (1995) work in Guyana.

However it is the qualities that the home visitor brings to the job rather than the background from which they come that ultimately appear to contribute more to their effectiveness. In particular, it is important that:

- *They have an empathy with the culture of the family.* Families are then more accepting and trusting of them.
- *They respond practically to the family's needs.* Parents should experience some immediate benefits from having a home visitor.
- *They try to involve all family members.* Mothers in particular have to fulfil many roles in developing countries. Grandparents, siblings and cousins can all be recruited to assist with the child with Down syndrome.
- *They empower families to be decision-makers.* They should share information and expertise freely with families so that they are empowered to make decisions and solve their problems.

Although the options for finding effective home visitors are available in most communities around the world, we should not underestimate the amount of effort which needs to be expended on recruiting suitable persons and the inevitable turnover which occurs with poorly paid or volunteer workers.

Parent associations

A second strategy for involving families is by bringing them together for regular meetings over a period of time. Such groups may develop into local associations for parents and friends. Indeed in most western countries, the formation of parent associations has been a major influence on the development of services. Often parent groups have grown out of the work begun by home visitors. They are also a powerful resource for educating local communities about disability. Such groups offer four advantages to parents.

Emotional support

Many parents feel isolated and shunned by society if they have a child with a marked disability. Having the opportunity to meet with others shows them that they are not alone and as their sense of solidarity grows they will be able to face the future more hopefully.

Advice and guidance

Families can draw on their own experience when offering advice to others. Their recommendations may be more credible than those offered by professionals who lack the day-to-day experience of living with a child who has a disability.

Advocacy on rights

An association can be a more effective promoter of rights than can individuals. The combined energies, expertise and experiences make it easier to develop and sustain a campaign of persuading communities and even government of the rights of people with a disability and their families.

Services for members

Groups can offer services to one another through cooperative endeavour. For example, parents may take it in turns to 'staff' a crèche or a day centre so that mothers can have some free time. Many associations have opened resource centres for their members where they can meet visiting specialists, obtain information, borrow toys and equipment, and attend income-generating activities.

Strategy 2: Mobilizing communities

The second strategy for creating more positive lifestyles for people with Down syndrome is to mobilize the community to act as a resource for their growth and development. The reasons are easily stated.

- Community services such as healthcare and schools need to be available to these children and their families. Experience shows however that often children with a disability are excluded either through ignorance or by intention.
- If young people with Down syndrome are to enjoy a full and decent life, then they cannot always remain at home. Communities offer opportunities for leisure and recreation, for making friends and developing relationships.
- In order to become economically self-reliant, young people with a disability need to find productive work beyond the family. Once again it is local communities that are best placed to respond to these needs.

However, few communities around the world are naturally disposed to becoming involved with people with a disability. Often it is the converse, with people holding negative perceptions based on fears and superstitions. The first task therefore is to educate communities about disability.

Disability awareness

Parent associations along with organizations for individuals with a disability have a particular contribution to make here. In Lesotho, for example, groups of parents have been trained to organize village gatherings where through songs, skits and talks they promote the rights of their child (McConkey, Mariga, Braadland and Mphole, 2000). Likewise, in Guyana volunteers from the Community Based Rehabilitation Programme organized puppet shows in schools and community centres to make pupils and communities more aware of the needs of this group. Other methods include the production of newsletters and poster campaigns along with the use of the media such as newspapers and radio to make people better informed about disability and more aware of what they can do to help (O'Toole, 1995).

Target groups

In all communities of the world, there are two groups of people who can be of particular help to families who have a child with a disability, namely, primary healthcare workers and teachers in nursery and primary schools. Both groups often lack experience and training in dealing with children who have Down syndrome. A priority is to ensure that information about disabilities in general and Down syndrome in particular is made available to them through their initial training courses or as part of their in-service training.

Training courses

The provision of training courses for community workers, teachers and even families is a relatively new concept in disability services. Unlike traditional college-based courses, community training has the following requirements.

- It should be locally available.
- The content should draw on family and community experiences and be applicable to those settings.
- Learning should take place through seeing and doing rather than by listening and reading. People with low academic attainments will thus learn better.
- Groups need to have a local person to lead them through the training courses.

The Community Based Rehabilitation Programme in Guyana has produced a number of training packages centred around specially made video programmes recorded in family and community settings. These programmes are shown in villages with a locally recruited person to act as course leader (O'Toole and McConkey, 1998).

Experienced community volunteers have organized local courses for various groups using specific training packages. For example, a training package on integrating children into mainstream schools has been used by a cadre of experienced community based rehabilitation (CBR) workers to provide a 20-hour training course for teachers from nursery and primary schools in their areas. Nearly 300 teachers participated in local courses in one year.

Likewise a training package giving basic health messages – *Facts for Life* – was presented by local CBR teams to over 4000 persons in the interior region of Guyana and two recently produced packages aimed at promoting the well-being and development of all children and hence preventing developmental disabilities – *A New Tomorrow* and *When There Is No Nursery School* – have been used with approximately 2000 persons.

Successful trainers

When we free our mind from the traditional image of 'trainers in disability services' we can begin to appreciate that the number of potential tutors could be very much greater if they were provided with suitable resource materials. Community staff, parents of people with disabilities, and people with disabilities themselves are but three groups who would be well motivated to undertake the task.

Experience in Guyana suggests that successful tutors tend to have the following attributes.

- They are very familiar with the local culture. If they are expatriate workers they need to have been in the country for five or more years.
- They may be trained and experienced professionals but they are able and willing to step outside their particular specialism to provide 'multi-disciplinary' training opportunities. Often they have been able to call on a network of contacts in other disciplines to supplement their knowledge and expertise.
- They are able communicators who form a ready rapport with the trainees.
- They are highly motivated to help people with disabilities and their families and to provide inspiration to others.
- Last, but by no means least, they have a clear vision of service goals and they have a detailed plan for bringing them about. Central to these

endeavours is their direct involvement in the training of workers and families.

Training outcomes

How do we judge the success of training? Traditionally training in rehabilitation has been focused on equipping people with knowledge and skills. However the training offered to communities and families should produce at least three other important outcomes.

*   It engenders positive attitudes and increases motivation to assist people with a disability.
*   It changes the behaviour of family members and the community towards people with a disability and increases their interactions with them.
*   It encourages the development of local services through the initiatives of local people and further promotes their capacity to be self-reliant.

Community forums

Finally, one promising development for sustaining community involvement has been the establishment of community forums made up of community leaders and workers, parents and people with disabilities. Their role is to plan and organize local services for children and adults with disabilities and to integrate these initiatives with other community development projects in the district or region.

Strategy 3: National policies

The third strategy for creating more positive lifestyles for all people with disabilities is through the development and implementation of national policies in key areas such as medical care, inclusive education and employment. The groundwork for this has been laid, in that nearly all world governments are signatories to two important Declarations of Rights.

The United Nations Declaration on the Rights of Disabled Persons (1975) states:

> Disabled persons whatever the origin, nature and seriousness of their handicaps and disabilities have the same fundamental rights as their fellow-citizens of the same age, which implies first and foremost the right to enjoy a decent life, as normal and as full as possible.
>
> (Article 3)

Likewise, the governments of the world have agreed that the same rights apply to all children irrespective of their impairments or environments. Hence the Convention on the Rights of the Child (UNICEF, 1990) states that:

Recognising the special needs of a disabled child, assistance . . . shall be provided to ensure that the disabled child has effective access to and receives education . . . conducive to the child achieving the fullest possible social integration and individual development.

(Article 23)

Both these declarations make clear how important it is for all citizens to participate fully in their community and for children especially to have the opportunity to grow into their culture, absorb its values and beliefs, and contribute to its development.

The age-old problem, though, is translating the rhetoric into practice. To that end, the United Nations produced a set of 'Standard Rules on the Equalization of Opportunities for Persons with Disabilities' (1994). The rules are intended to form an instrument for nation states to use in formulating policy and practices that ensure that the rights of children with disabilities and their families are upheld.

The rules are grouped thematically and cover areas such as medical care, support services, education, employment and economic policies. For example, Rule Seven in the Employment section states:

The aim should always be for persons with disabilities to obtain employment in the open labour market. For persons with disabilities whose needs cannot be met in open employment, small units of sheltered or supported employment may be an alternative. It is important that the quality of such programmes be assessed in terms of their relevance and sufficiency in providing opportunities for persons with disabilities to gain employment in the labour market.

The Standard Rules provide essential information for lobbyists seeking to influence national legislation and policies.

Influencing policy

As noted earlier, disability will *not* be a priority for government expenditure in most developing countries. It is therefore unrealistic to expect them to directly fund services. Rather, the energies of lobbyists are better directed at encouraging governments to set the context in which appropriate services can grow and develop. This means:

- Enacting legislation to safeguard the rights of people with disabilities. Two areas have been the focus of international lobbying: the right to education, and the right to equal job opportunities.
- Defining the government's aspirations as to the sorts of services they would like to see made available in the country for people with disabilities. Such statements have usually emerged from a process of systematic consultation with all interested parties and are updated through the

formation of government-sponsored bodies, such as a National Council for Disability.

- Assigning ministerial responsibility for disability issues, either within a single ministry, or by setting up an inter-ministerial group. This should make sure that a coordinated approach develops across interested ministries while at the same time ensuring that disability issues are brought to the attention of all ministers. Parallel structures need to be developed for local government.

- Developing national standards for services and evolving mechanisms to ensure that these standards are maintained. This would apply in the first instance to services provided by government, such as education, health and social welfare services as well as those by voluntary groups.

- The training of significant professionals in government service, namely, teachers, nurses and doctors, should embrace disability issues.

Sad to say, the majority of governments have yet to embark on such programmes but much can be learnt from the experiences of those that have done so.

Alliances of common concern

In any democracy, governments are more susceptible to influence when it comes from large, representative groups with an agreed plan of action. Arguably one of the biggest shortcomings of the disability movement worldwide has been the fragmentation that exists not only across different impairments but also among parents and disabled activists claiming to represent the same group. Although there is much they can and do achieve for individual families or local communities, when it comes to influencing national policy, it is essential to form alliances with other like-minded groups.

This need not mean losing one's autonomy to act independently on other issues or imply a take-over by a more powerful agency. Rather the alliance is an opportunity to unite on particular issues that affect all members and to lobby for specific actions that will ultimately produce a better quality of life for all those with disabilities. Down Syndrome Associations have been formed in many countries of the world. Too often, I fear, they stand alone from other groups as they seek particular benefits for their members. I trust that with maturity will come a growing confidence that will enable them to take their rightful place in alliances with other groups to lobby for early intervention, education and employment for all children born with impairments.

Where should the focus of activity be?

There are three priority areas in which efforts to assist people with Down syndrome who live in developing countries must be focused (McConkey, 1996). They are the three 'E's of:

- Early intervention from the first months of life;
- Education, ideally from nursery school and through all the years of primary schooling;
- Employment, either as productive members of their family or in some form of income generating activity.

Early intervention

The growth and development of infants with Down syndrome needs to be stimulated through regular exercises, activities and involvement in family routines. The impact of early intervention programmes is well documented in affluent countries (Farran, 1990) and there is every reason to believe that similar interventions will be equally effective in poorer countries despite the extra economic and social stresses these families face (Zinkin and McConachie, 1995).

Education

Although the world's nations aspire to making education available for all children, a recent review paper prepared for the World Education Forum held in Senegal in April 2000, estimated that 113 million children have no access to primary education; particularly disadvantaged were girls, working children and those with special needs. In affluent countries, children with Down syndrome have traditionally attended special schools but increasingly parents are opting for regular schooling with extra supports. In the developing world, few special schools exist and for most countries this is an unaffordable option even if it was thought desirable. Hence the only opportunity for many children with Down syndrome to be educated is by attending the local school (Hegarty, 1993). For these families, inclusive education is not an option but a necessity.

Employment

Disability and poverty are often first cousins throughout the world but more especially in poorer countries where there are no social security benefits. Any member of the family who is not productive is therefore a drain on family resources. Hence as far as possible, children with Down syndrome need to become self-reliant in their personal care and to be able to undertake jobs around the house, such as water fetching, in order that the family workload is shared. It is better still if the young people can play a part in income generation, perhaps by assisting on the family farm or business or by holding down a job with local employers (Neufeldt, 1995).

The goals outlined above for early intervention, education and employment are not easily or quickly achievable and, sadly, they are more realistic for some children and their families than others. However they are realizable through the three strategies of family involvement, community mobilization and the promotion of rights.

A dream come true?

Much of the foregoing will seem like dreams as these words are read in developing countries by families and indeed many professional workers such as teachers and doctors. Likewise, the readers from a previous generation in affluent countries would also have considered them to be fanciful imaginings. But as this volume and the World Congress from which it emanated demonstrated, many of these dreams have become a reality in parts of the world.

Down syndrome is not a disaster for either the person or the family but rather a road less travelled. It is a journey that increasingly is becoming better signposted with improved facilities en route and one that brings rich rewards to those who venture forth in hope and with determination. As is often the case in the developing world, the roads are ill-defined and filled with potholes but through the efforts of dedicated parents and professionals, there too a highway for people with Down syndrome is also starting to take shape. This chapter is dedicated to their efforts.

References

Brohier B (1995) Funding services. In O'Toole BJ, McConkey R (Eds) Innovations in Developing Countries for People with Disabilities. Chorley, Lancs: Lisieux Hall Publications. pp 227-42.

Coleridge P (1993) Disability, Liberation and Development. Oxford: Oxfam.

Farran DC (1990) Effects of intervention with disadvantaged and disabled children: a decade review. In Meisels SJ, Shonkoff JP (Eds) Handbook of Early Childhood Intervention. Cambridge: Cambridge University Press. pp 501-39.

Gallagher JJ (1990) The family as a focus for intervention. In Meisels SJ, Shonkoff JP (Eds) Handbook of Early Childhood Intervention. Cambridge: Cambridge University Press. pp 540-59.

Hegarty (1993) Education of children with disabilities. In Mittler P, Brouillette R, Harris D (Eds) World Yearbook of Education 1993: Special Needs Education. London: Kogan Page. pp 16-28.

Helander E (1993) Prejudice and Dignity: An Introduction to Community Based Rehabilitation. Geneva: UNDP.
Jaffer R, Jaffer R (1990) The WHO–CBR approach: programme or ideology? Some lessons from the CBR experience in Punjab, Pakistan. In Thorburn M, Marfo K (Eds) Practical Approaches to Childhood Disability in Developing Countries: Insights From Experience and Research. St John's: Memorial University of Newfoundland. pp 277-92.
McConkey R (1996) Down syndrome and developing countries. In Stratford B, Gunn P (Eds) New Approaches to Down Syndrome. London: Cassell. pp 451-96.
McConkey R, Mariga L, Braadland N, Mphole P (2000) Parents as trainers about disability in low income countries. International Journal of Disability, Development and Education 47: 309-17.
McGlade B, Acquino R (1995) Mothers of disabled children as CBR workers. In O'Toole BJ, McConkey R (Eds) Innovations in Developing Countries for People with Disabilities. Chorley, Lancs: Lisieux Hall Publications. pp 183-98.
Neufeldt A (1995) Self-directed employment and economic independence in low-income countries. In O'Toole BJ, McConkey R (Eds) Innovations in Developing Countries for People with Disabilities. Chorley, Lancs: Lisieux Hall Publications. pp 161-82.
O'Toole B (1995) Mobilising communities. In O'Toole BJ, McConkey R (Eds) Innovations in Developing Countries for People with Disabilities. Chorley, Lancs: Lisieux Hall Publications. pp 85-104.
O'Toole B, McConkey R (1998) A national training strategy for personnel working in developing countries: an example from Guyana. International Journal of Rehabilitation Research 21: 311-21.
Schwartz DB (1992) Crossing the River: Creating a Conceptual Revolution in Community and Disability. Cambridge, MA: Brookline Books.
Thorburn MJ (1990) Training community workers for early detection, assessment and intervention. In Thorburn M, Marfo K (Eds) Practical Approaches to Childhood Disability in Developing Countries: Insights From Experience and Research. St John's: Memorial University of Newfoundland.
UNICEF (1990) First Call for Children. New York: UNICEF
United Nations (1975) The Rights of Disabled Persons. New York: United Nations.
United Nations (1994) The Standard Rules on the Equalization of Opportunities for Persons with Disabilities. New York: United Nations.
Werner D (1987) Disabled Village Children. Palo Alto, CA: Hesperian Foundation.
White BL (1979) The First Three Years of Life. New York: Avon Books.
Zinkin P, McConachie H (1995) Disabled Children and Developing Countries. London: Mackeith Press.

Index

whole language approaches, literacy development, 83–84, 85
Woodcock Reading Mastery Test–Revised, 89
working memory, *see* short-term memory
work placement, *see* employment
World Education Forum, 207
World Health Organization, 199

writing
joint construction of texts, 88
LATCH-ON, 88–89
representations of people with Down syndrome, 8
work placement, 141

Xin, Y. P., 82